SUZY PRUDDEN'S
SPOT
REDUCING
PROGRAM

SUZY PRUDDEN'S SPOT REDUCING PROGRAM

BY SUZY PRUDDEN AND JEFFREY SUSSMAN

PHOTOGRAPHS BY MORT ENGEL

WORKMAN PUBLISHING, NEW YORK

BOOKS BY SUZY PRUDDEN & JEFFREY SUSSMAN

Creative Fitness For Baby & Child
Suzy Prudden's Family Fitness Book
Fit For Life
See How They Run

Library of Congress Cataloging in Publication Data

Prudden, Suzy.
  Suzy Prudden's Spot reducing program.
  1. Reducing exercises. I. Sussman, Jeffrey, joint author. II. Title. III. Title: Spot reducing program.
RA781.6.P78   613.7′1   79-64784
ISBN 0-89480-115-5
ISBN 0-89480-114-7 pbk.

Cover and book design: Charles Kreloff
Suzy Prudden's leotards by Capezio Ballet Makers

Manufactured in the United States of America
First printing October 1979

10 9 8 7 6 5 4

Workman Publishing Company, Inc.
1 West 39 Street
New York, New York 10018

DEDICATION

There are many people who have helped us both in words and deeds. This book is dedicated to them as well as to our son, Robby. To Joseph Greenberg, Peter Grunebaum, Gula V. Hirschland, Herbert and Ethel Hirschland, and Flora Mack.

And, as always, in memory of our fathers: Richard Hirschland and Robert Sussman.

ACKNOWLEDGEMENTS

We have never met a publishing company whose staff worked with such dedication and enthusiasm as those at Workman. In particular, we are grateful to Peter Workman for his sweet rationality, to the diligent editorial efforts of Sally Kovalchick and Carol Wallace, and finally we are grateful to the aesthetic sensibilities of Charles Kreloff, who designed this book. There are many others whose talents have been of inestimable value, but we cannot list everyone in the employ of Workman.

CONTENTS

INTRODUCTION

Spot reducing is a program of exercises designed to tighten, tone, and reduce specific parts of your body: arms, shoulders, breasts, waist, stomach, hips, thighs, fanny, calves, and even ankles. It is an effective method for reshaping your figure to make you look as attractive as you possibly can.

Overall weight loss, while slimming most of your body, may fail to eliminate fat that collects around rarely or improperly used muscles. Spot reducing concentrates on these particular problem areas, strengthening and streamlining the muscles involved, to ensure a flab-free, well-toned body.

This book is divided into sets of exercises, each concentrating on one area of the body. The exercises in each section have been chosen because they work on those muscles in isolation, strengthening and toning them in order to trim undesirable bulges. Since they are arranged within the section to give your muscles a complete workout without straining them, you should do all the exercises in the order given.

Many people will want to concentrate on more than one figure problem: hips and thighs, waist and stomach, ankles and calves—difficulties in these areas seem to go together. If you want to work on more than one part of your body, simply combine a number of spot reducing exercises. If you want to reshape your entire body, that too is possible; do all the exercises for a thorough workout.

Performing these movements correctly and conscientiously will produce noticeable improvement after only three weeks of daily exercising. After that time, you should change over to the maintenance routines for your problem areas. In most cases, the number of repetitions for each exercise will increase. The maintenance section at the back of the book, however, will tell you which exercises from each section will maintain the improvement you've made. Each maintenance program is designed to take no more than twenty minutes.

Remember: spot reducing will reshape particular parts of your body—and that is *all* it will do. It is not a cardiovascular exercise, which quickens the pulse and the heartbeat, nor is it a substitute for weight control. If your flabby areas are caused by excess pounds, you must lose weight before you can see improvement. And although exercising can help to speed this process, the only way to lose weight is by sensible eating.

YOUR EXERCISE SESSION

These exercises incorporate simple movements that do not demand great skill or experience. Though some are more strenuous than others, none should be beyond your capability. You should feel your muscles working, contracting and relaxing, but you should never strain them. Above all, you should never feel pain. Pain is a warning signal from your body that you are doing something wrong, and that you should stop immediately. The exercises in this book were carefully prepared to give your muscles a workout without injuring them.

Since a daily routine is essential, you should make exercising as pleasant as possible. Music can be a marvelous addition to exercise sessions: not only is it fun to listen to, but it will help make the movements of the exercises rhythmic and regular. You might prefer to do your exercises on a mat if you find a bare floor uncomfortable. If you choose to use a rug instead, be careful that it doesn't slip on a wood floor. You don't have to wear a leotard, but you should wear loose clothing that does not limit your movements. And, before you begin, you may want to measure the parts of your body you plan to trim. As you see those inches melting away, you'll be encouraged to stick with your reducing and maintenance programs.

Perhaps the most important feature of spot reducing is that it need not take a lot of time. You can devote as little as twenty minutes each day to working on your specific problems. And if you're already in good condition, you may want to spend an additional ten minutes daily to preserve the fitness of your entire body.

The book also includes a section of flexibility exercises. While these do not work to reduce specific areas of flab, they should be an integral part of your exercise program. They will make your muscles supple and limber, and less susceptible to injury. Your muscles will become long and lean rather than short and bulky. Moreover, as you become more flexible, both your exercise routine and your everyday movements will become more graceful.

THE PROCEDURES

Before you begin an exercise, read the instructions carefully, familiarizing yourself with all the movements involved in the sequence. Concentrate on doing the exercise correctly and following the photographs as closely as possible. Do not strain your muscles; work only to the point at which you are comfortable. Move smoothly, because jerky motions are likely to cause discomfort.

When an exercise calls for your arms and legs to be stretched out, really reach with them; extending them as far as possible causes best results. And concentrate on keeping your stomach pulled in and your fanny tightened. In a short time, and with a minimum amount of effort, you'll find yourself the proud owner of the body you've always wanted.

9

ARMS

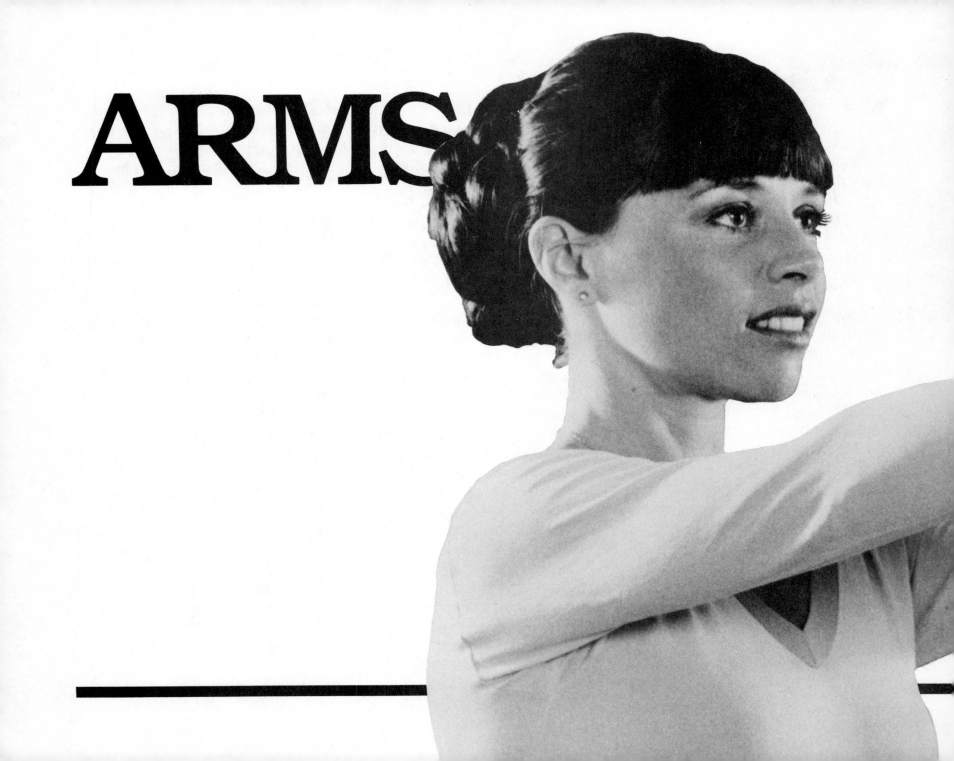

Most women neglect to exercise their arms. How many regularly lift heavy loads or use their arms for strenuous and frequent exercise? And while troubled by heavy thighs or a big stomach, they don't give a thought to seeing that their arms are in shape. Yet upper arms are often the first part of the body to sag, no matter how slim or fit a woman might be.

The biceps and triceps muscles are the ones to exercise in order to firm sagging arms. The following routines strengthen and tone these muscles without making them large and bulky.

While you do the routines, stretch and twist your arms as far as possible to make your muscles long and lean.

Some of the exercises tone and strengthen the forearm as well as the upper arm, and will ensure firm and graceful limbs.

TABLE LIFT

This exercise is especially good for strengthening and toning your upper arms. Be sure your arms are straight throughout the sequence.

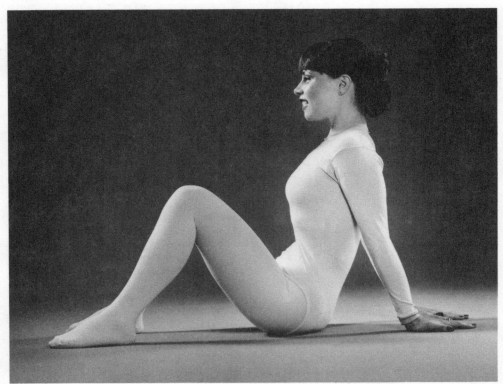

To Reduce: repeat 4 times

Maintenance: repeat 8 times

1

Sit on the floor with your legs slightly apart, knees bent, and feet flat on the floor. Place the palms of your hands on the floor several inches behind your fanny, being sure to keep your fingers pointing away from your body.

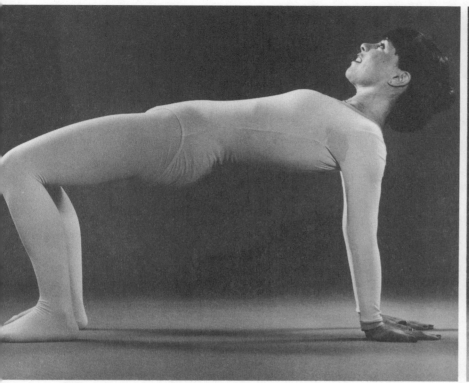

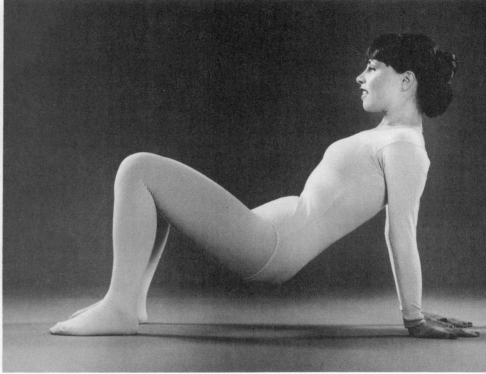

2

Lift your fanny and push
your entire torso into the
air so it is parallel to the
floor. Do not bend at the
waist; your body should
form a straight line
between knees and
shoulders. Hold the
raised position for 6 seconds.
Keep your arms straight.

3

Slowly lowering your
fanny, return to the
original position.

BELLOWS PUSH-UP

Though less strenuous than the conventional push-up, this exercise works well to strengthen the upper arms.

To Reduce: repeat 4 times

Maintenance: repeat 8 times

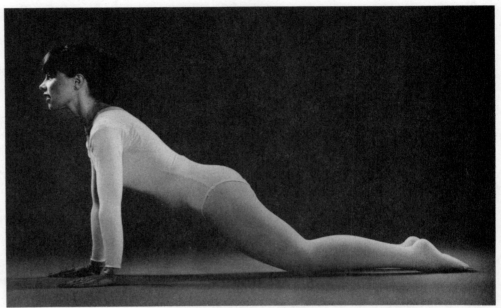

1

Beginning down on your hands and knees, move your hands forward slightly with the palms flat and the fingers pointing ahead of you. Push your weight forward so that your arms are straight with your hands under your shoulders and the fronts of your thighs form a 45-degree angle with the floor.

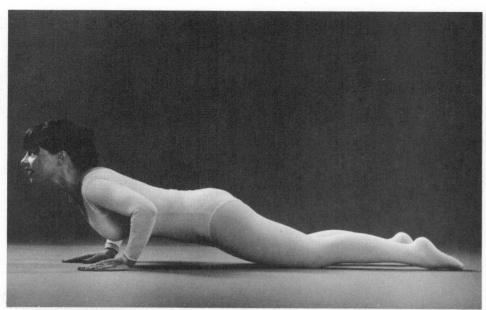

2

While counting slowly to four, bend your arms and gradually lower your torso almost to the floor, keeping your back and neck as straight as possible.

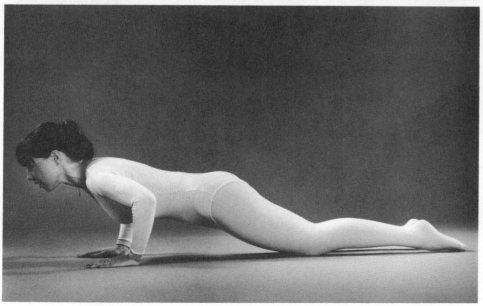

3

Without allowing your torso to touch the floor, raise your body by straightening your arms, again to the count of four.

LOWERING RAMP

While doing this exercise, try to think of your body as a straight line from head to toe. Don't allow your stomach to sag, and keep your fanny tucked in.

To Reduce: repeat 4 times

Maintenance: repeat 8 times

You may be able to do a conventional push-up after several weeks; if so, work your way up to 4 to 6 push-ups each day.

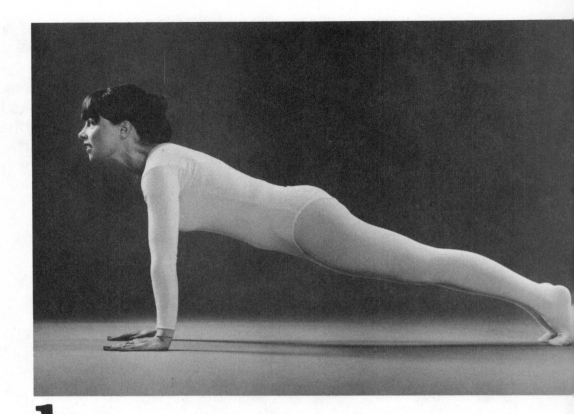

1

Assume the conventional push-up position: body straight, supported by straight arms and the balls of your feet.

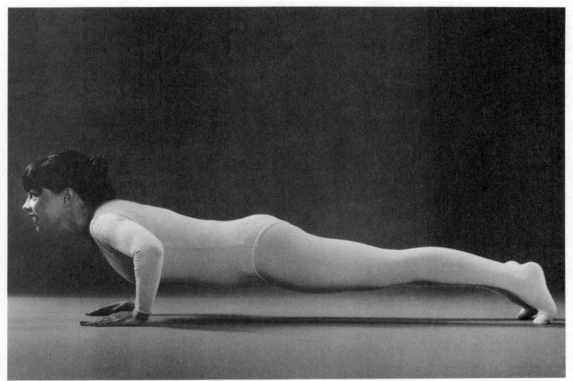

2

While counting slowly to
five, lower your body
by bending your elbows.
Do not bend at the
waist. Be sure not to let
your body rest on the
floor until you have
reached the count of five.

TAKING OFF

This exercise is excellent for trimming the inside of the upper arm. For best results, keep the circular motions of your arms small and smooth. Be sure to turn your arms as far as possible.

To Reduce: repeat sequence (8 circles backward and 8 circles forward) twice

Maintenance: the same

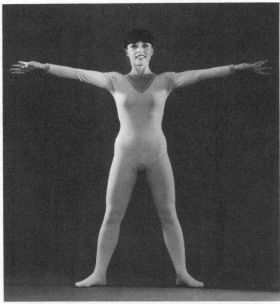

1

Stand straight with your feet apart and arms stretched out to the side at shoulder height. Turn the palms of your hands up, then back as far as possible, keeping your arms straight.

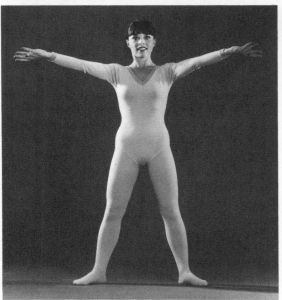

2

With your palms turned back, rotate your arms in a backward motion, making 8 full circles.

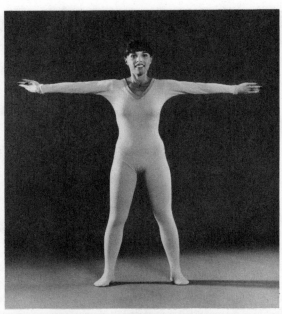

3

Keeping your arms stretched out to the side, turn your palms down, then back and up so they face the ceiling.

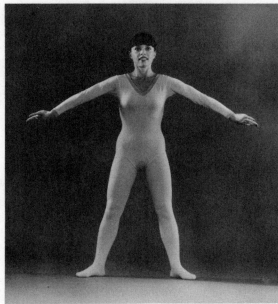

4

Holding this position, rotate your arms in a forward circle 8 times.

RAISING THE FLAG

One of the most strenuous exercises for upper arms, this involves supporting most of your weight on one arm. As your arms grow stronger, however, you'll find it easier to do.

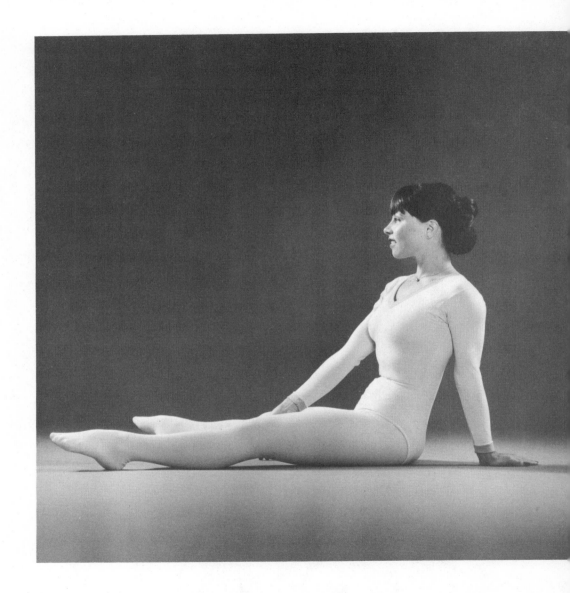

To Reduce: repeat 4 times on each side

Maintenance: repeat 8 times on each side

1

Sit on the floor with your legs extended, slightly apart, and with feet pointed. Place the palm of your left hand flat on the floor behind your fanny, and relax your right arm in front of you.

2

Using your left arm for leverage, push your torso up from the floor so your body forms a straight line between feet and shoulders. At the same time, in one continuous motion, bring your right arm up to form a straight line with your left arm. Hold this position for 3 seconds, then lower your torso and resume the original position.

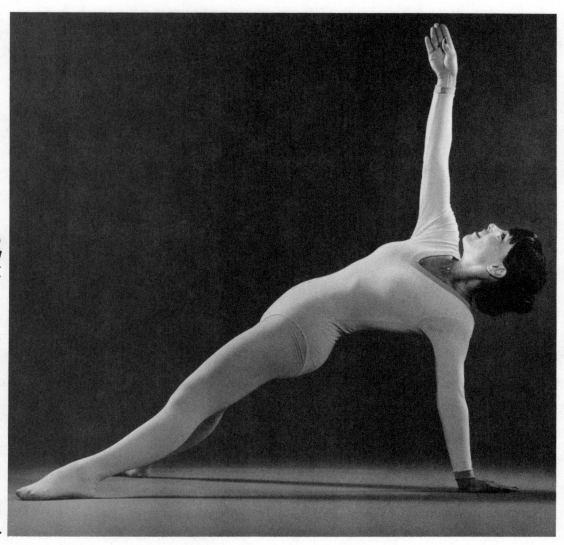

TENNIS BALL SQUEEZE

This simple but effective exercise will improve the shape of your forearms and strengthen your grip. If you have only one ball, exercise one hand at a time.

To Reduce: repeat 8 times

Maintenance: repeat 16 times or as often as you wish

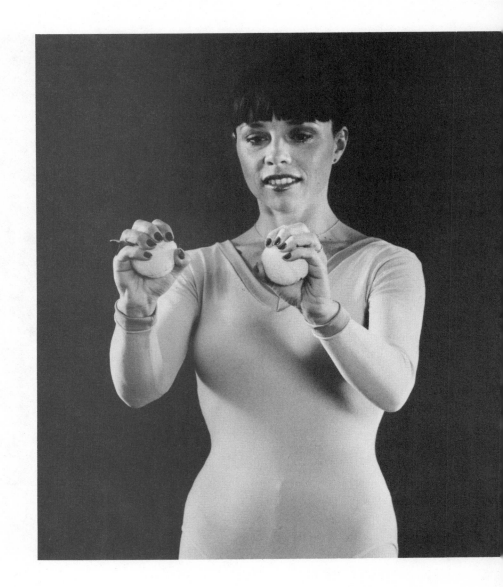

1

Hold a tennis ball (or rubber ball) in each hand, grasping it with your fingers. Your elbows should be bent.

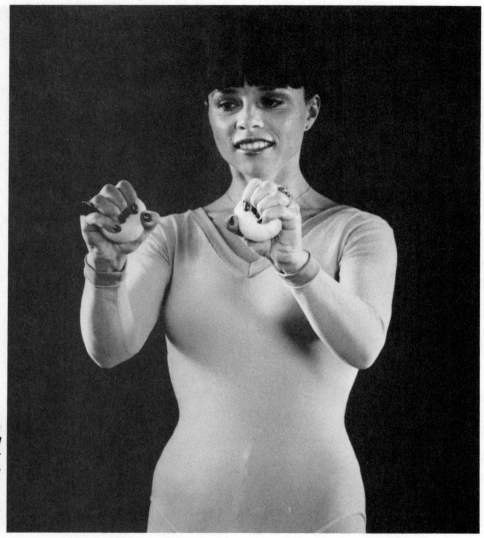

2

Squeeze the two balls as hard as you can for 3 seconds, then relax your grip.

FEELING IN THE DARK

In this exercise, it is important to keep the arms taut. Be sure that only your forearms twist while your shoulders remain still.

To Reduce: complete sequence once

Maintenance: the same

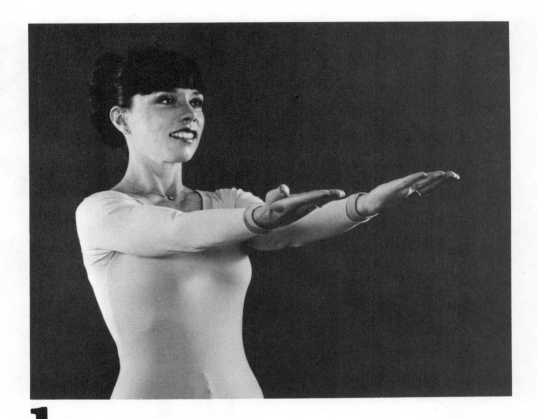

1

Stand straight with your feet slightly apart and your arms extended in front at shoulder height. Turn your palms up, making sure the undersides of your forearms are also turned upward.

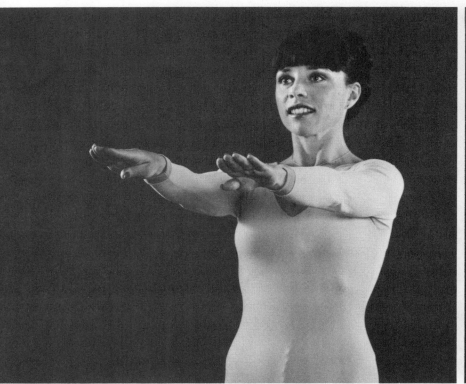

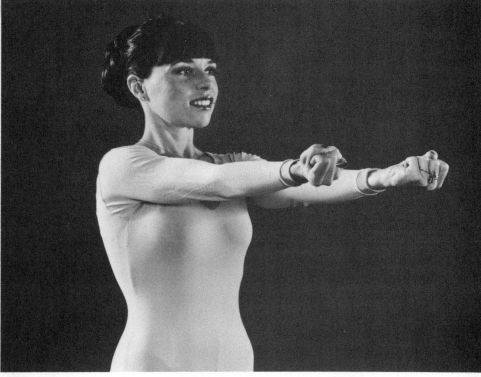

2

Stretching your arms
forward and keeping your
elbows still, turn your
palms down, then up
again. Repeat 12 times.

3

With your palms down,
make your hands into
fists and turn them up,
then down, 12 times in
the same manner.

FIGHTING YOURSELF

This isometric exercise can be done anywhere, at any time of day and shapes forearms as well as upper arms.

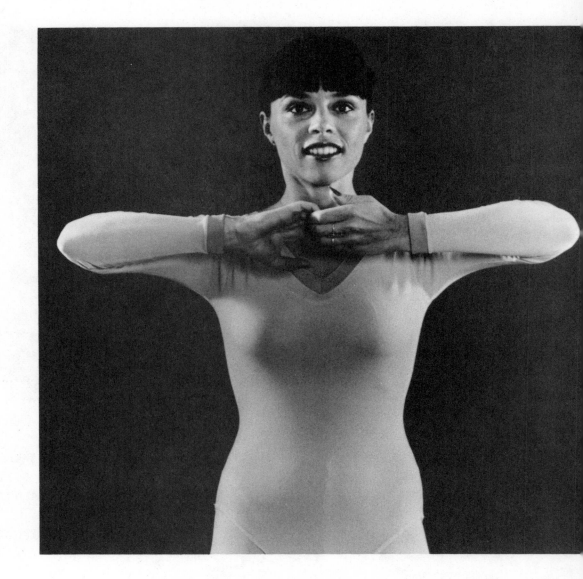

To Reduce: repeat sequence 8 times

Maintenance: repeat sequence 16 times

1

Stand straight with your feet slightly apart and your fingers clasped in front of your chest. Pull with your arms as hard as you can away from your clasped fingers and hold the pulling position for 3 seconds.

2

Press your hands against each other and push them as hard as you can into the hand press. Hold the pushing position for 3 seconds.

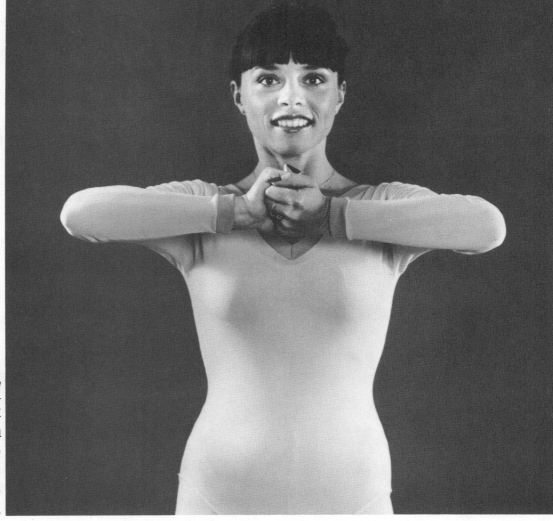

SHOULDERS
& BREASTS

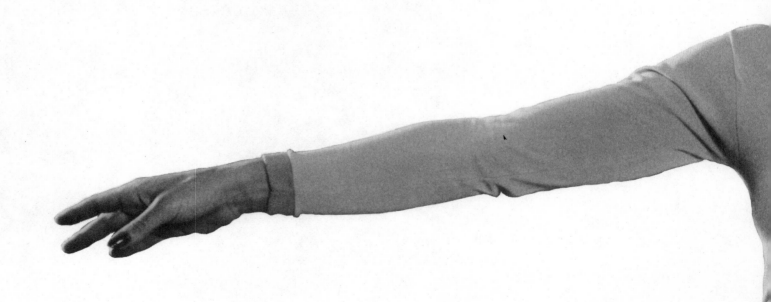

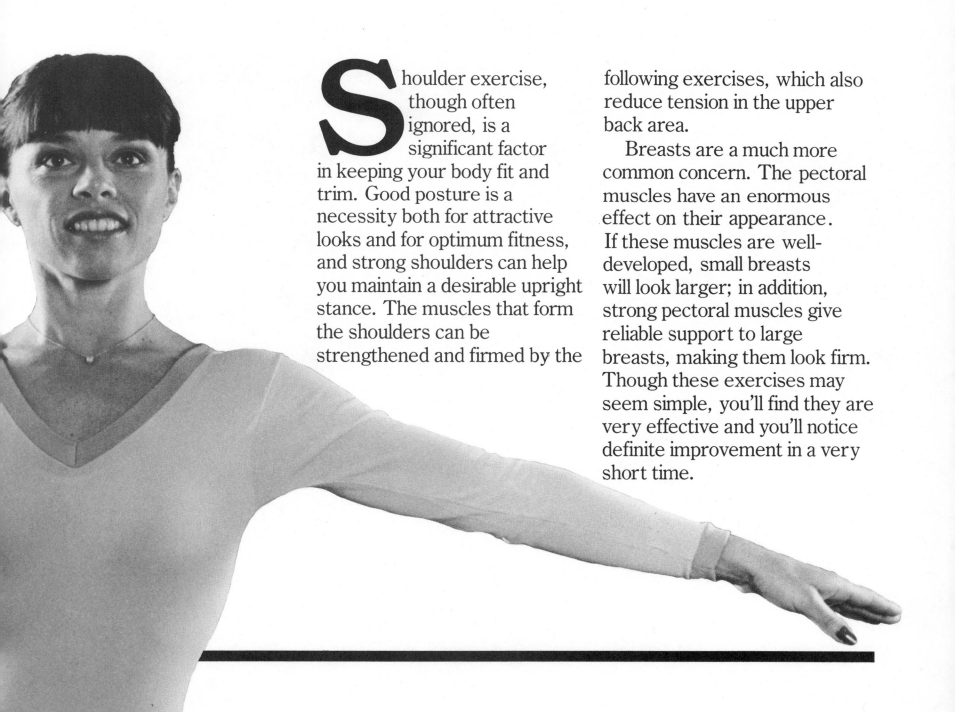

Shoulder exercise, though often ignored, is a significant factor in keeping your body fit and trim. Good posture is a necessity both for attractive looks and for optimum fitness, and strong shoulders can help you maintain a desirable upright stance. The muscles that form the shoulders can be strengthened and firmed by the following exercises, which also reduce tension in the upper back area.

Breasts are a much more common concern. The pectoral muscles have an enormous effect on their appearance. If these muscles are well-developed, small breasts will look larger; in addition, strong pectoral muscles give reliable support to large breasts, making them look firm. Though these exercises may seem simple, you'll find they are very effective and you'll notice definite improvement in a very short time.

THE SHRUG

This exercise exaggerates a common gesture to give your shoulders a workout. It is also effective in relieving tension in the upper back area.

To Reduce: repeat sequence 8 times

Maintenance: repeat sequence 24 times (may be done in 3 sessions throughout the day)

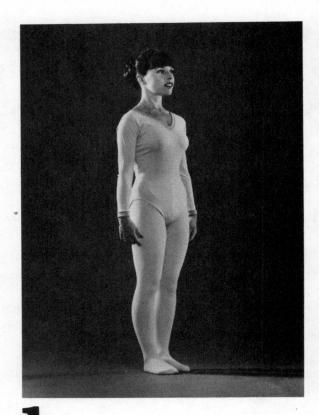

1

Stand straight with your feet together and your arms relaxed at your sides.

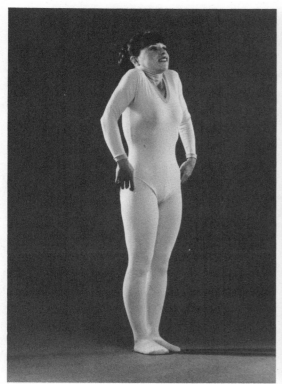

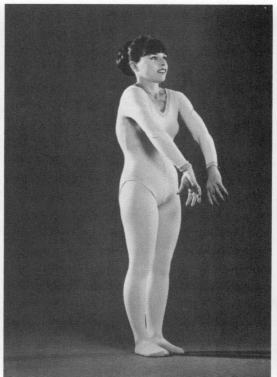

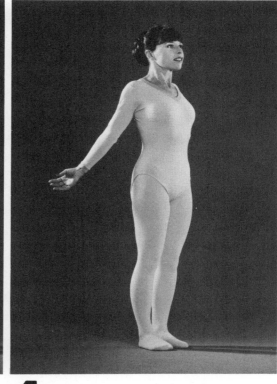

2

Lift your shoulders
straight up as far as
possible, as if to touch
them to your ears, then
lower them to the resting
position. Keep your body
still except for the
shoulder movement.

3

Round your shoulders
and push them forward,
again without moving the
rest of the body.

4

Push your shoulders back
as far as you can. Return
to the resting position.

SEXY SHOULDERS

By rotating your shoulders, you take The Shrug a step farther. This exercise is also good for relieving tension, especially after long periods of sitting still.

To Reduce: repeat sequence 4 times

Maintenance: repeat sequence 8 times

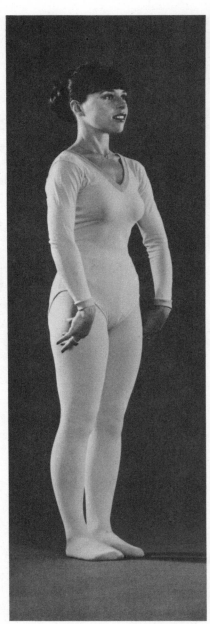

1

Stand straight with your feet together and your arms relaxed at your sides. Begin a rotating motion by rounding your shoulders forward.

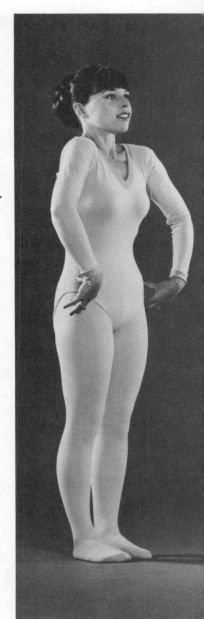

2

Lift your
shoulders up
toward your
ears.

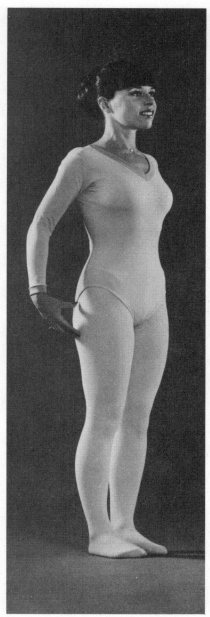

3

Stretch your
shoulders back
as far as
possible, then
lower them to
the resting
position.

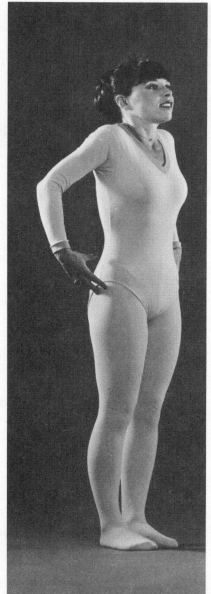

4

Reverse the
direction of the
exercise: move
your shoulders
back, then up
toward your
ears, then
forward.

33

SHOULDERS AND BREASTS

"T"-TWIST

The success of this exercise depends on stretching and twisting your arms as far as possible. It is excellent for trimming shoulders—and upper arms.

To Reduce: repeat sequence 8 times

Maintenance: repeat sequence 16 times

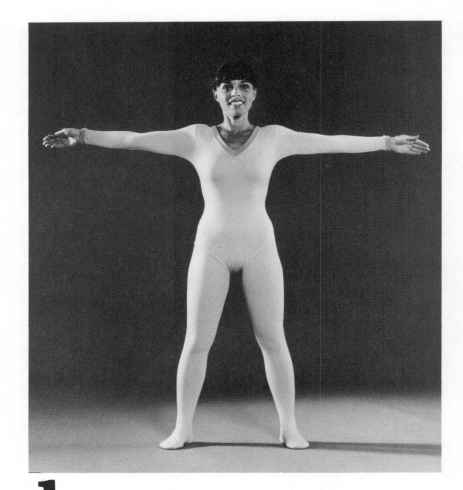

1

Stand with your feet apart and your arms stretched out to the side at shoulder height, palms of your hands facing front.

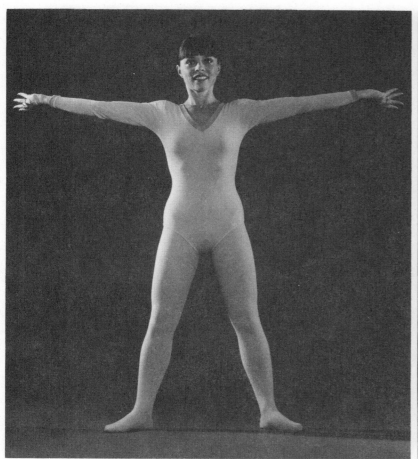

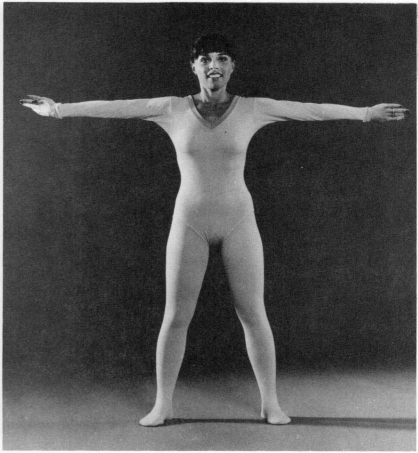

2

Keeping your arms
extended, turn your
palms up, then back as
far as possible. Your
shoulders should turn
slightly backward.

3

Turn your palms down,
then back, so that your
thumbs are pointing
behind you. Your shoulders
should turn slightly forward.
Do not bend your arms.

SHOULDERS AND BREASTS

THE NON-AQUATIC SWIM

This exercise tones both the shoulders and the upper arms. As you "swim," reach with your arms for best results. Keep your back flat and your legs straight. Your head and back should form a straight line.

To Reduce: complete sequence once

Maintenance: repeat sequence twice

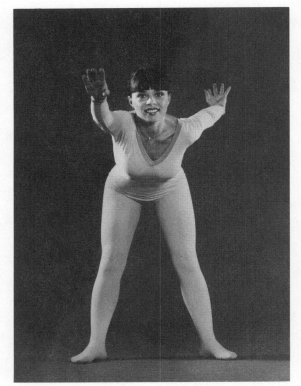

1

Standing with your legs straight and feet apart, bend forward at the hips so your torso is parallel to the floor. Stretch your right arm forward and your left arm back, both at shoulder height.

36

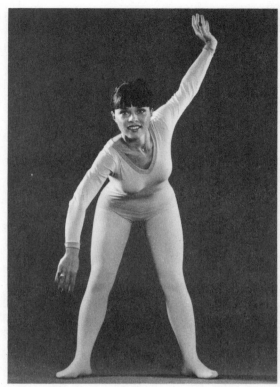

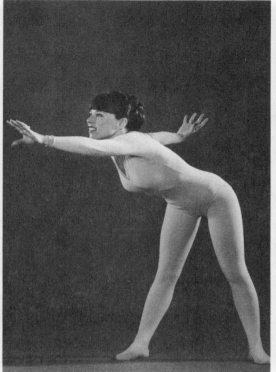

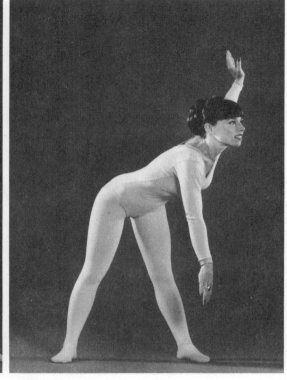

2

Rotate your arms in alternating circles, as if you were swimming. Keep your arms straight. Make 8 full circles with each arm.

3

Lean over your right leg and rotate your arms in the same manner. Make 8 full circles with each arm. Remember to keep your legs straight.

4

Lean over your left leg and make 8 more full circles with each arm. Return to the original position for 8 final rotations with each arm.

BUTTERFLY SALUTE

In making half-circles with your arms, be sure to use a smooth motion. Keep your stomach muscles tight and don't arch your back when you swing your arm behind you.

To Reduce: complete sequence once

Maintenance: the same

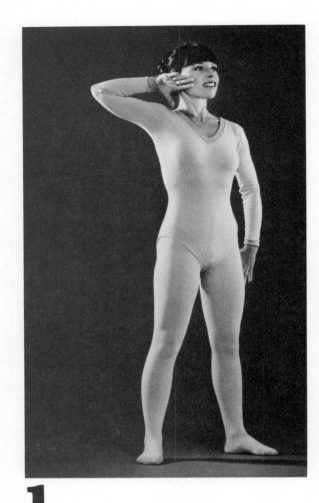

1

Stand straight with your feet apart and arms relaxed at your sides. Bring your right elbow up and back. Keep your right palm facing out, fingers against your cheek.

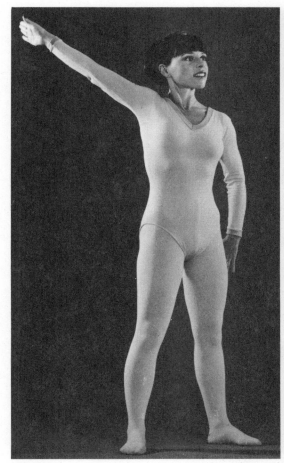 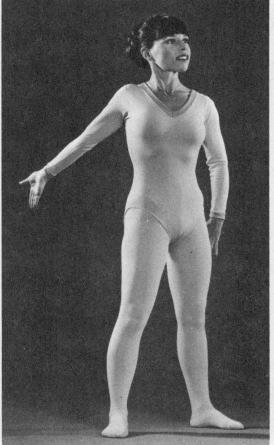 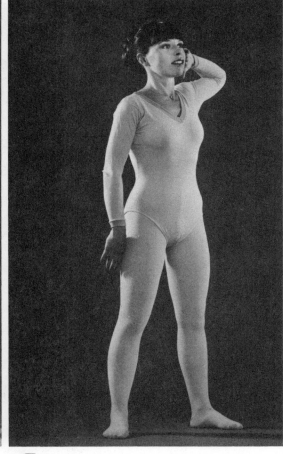

2

Straighten your right arm so it reaches up and in back of you.

3

Make a half-circle with your arm, bringing it downward to rest at your side.

4

Repeat with your left arm. Alternating arms, make 16 half-circles (8 with each arm). Repeat 4 final times, using both arms at once.

SHOULDERS AND BREASTS

WINGING IT

Once you become familiar with this exercise, you should be able to do it smoothly, without pausing. Keep your stomach and fanny muscles tightened throughout, and be careful not to arch your back.

To Reduce: repeat sequence 16 times

Maintenance: repeat sequence 24 times

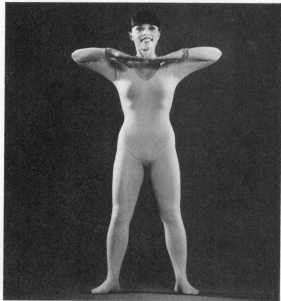

1

Stand straight with your feet apart and bend your arms at shoulder level, letting your fingers meet in front of your chest. Your palms should face the floor.

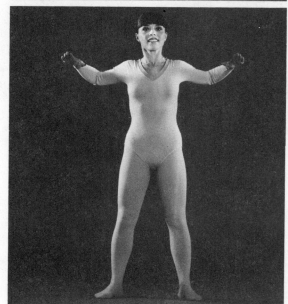

2

Move your arms back from the shoulder, keeping them bent so your elbows point behind you.

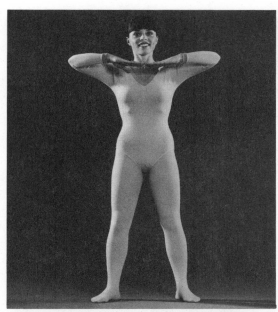

3

Bring your arms forward so your fingertips meet in front of you.

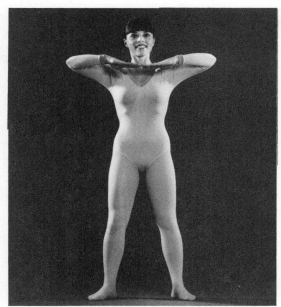

5

Return your arms to the original bent position, palms down, fingertips touching.

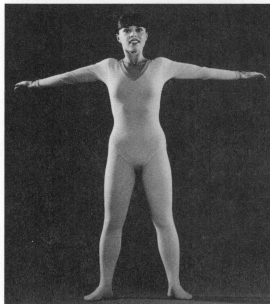

4

Turn your palms up toward the ceiling, then swing your arms out and back, straightening your elbows. Your arms should be outstretched, palms up, at shoulder height.

STAR DIVING

This exercise looks simple, but it is enormously effective in lifting the bust. Do not thrust your head forward or arch your back during this exercise.

To Reduce: repeat 12 times

Maintenance: repeat 16 times

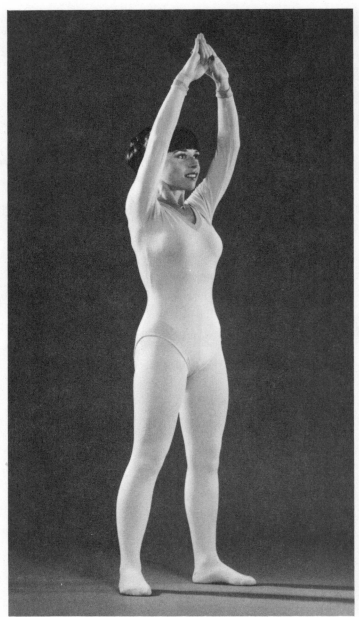

1
Stand straight with your feet apart and your arms extended above your head. Clasp your hands.

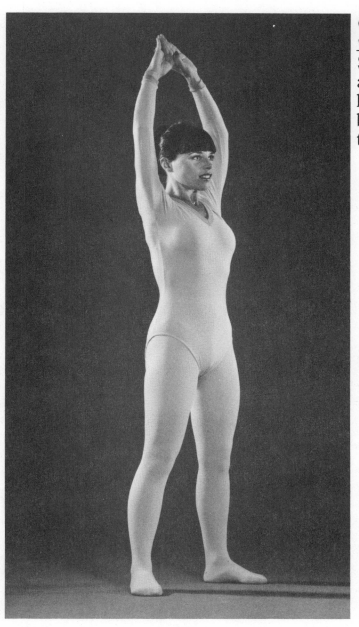

2

Stretch your arms back as far as you can while keeping them and your body straight. Return to the original position.

SHOULDERS AND BREASTS

TOWEL TUG

The purpose of this exercise is to develop and strengthen your pectoral muscles, which support your breasts. Remember to keep your stomach pulled in.

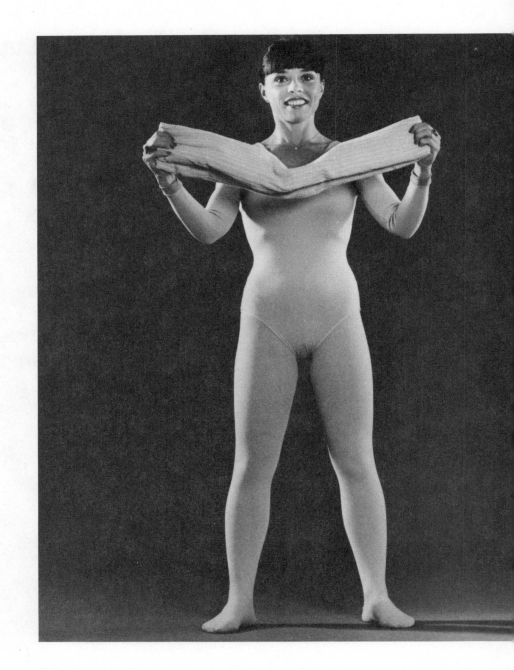

To Reduce: repeat 16 times

Maintenance: repeat 24 times

1

Stand with your feet apart, holding a small towel in front of you with one hand at each end. Your elbows should be bent and hands raised to shoulder height.

2

Maintaining the position of your upper arms, pull both ends of the towel as hard as possible until it is stretched taut. Hold this position for 3 seconds, then relax the tension on the towel.

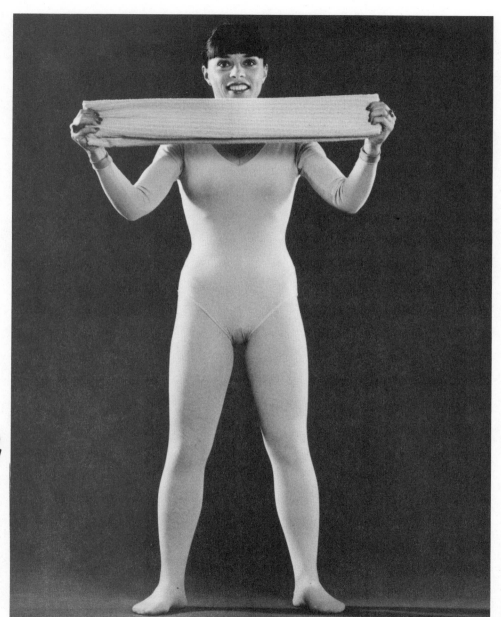

DOWEL DIP

This exercise is excellent for lifting your breasts, as well as for toning your midriff and waist. A broomstick can be used in place of a dowel, but be sure your hands are 3 feet apart. Do not lean forward or arch your back as you bend to the side.

To Reduce: repeat sequence 4 times

Maintenance: repeat sequence 8 times

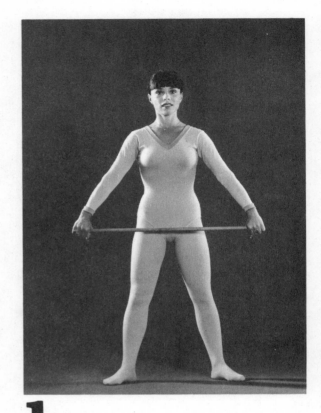

1

Stand with your feet apart and your legs straight. With hands 3 feet apart, hold a dowel in front of you just below your hips.

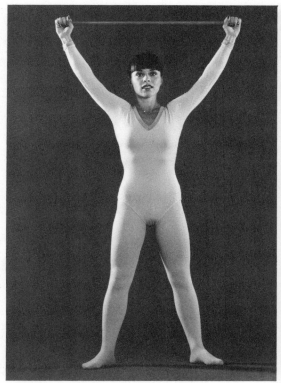

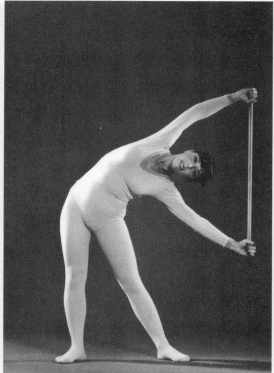

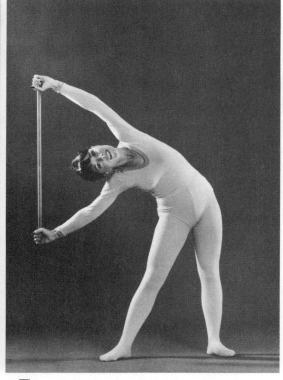

2

Raise your hands over your head, keeping your arms straight.

3

Bend your torso as far as you can to one side and bounce 4 times. Do not lean forward. After a week or two, you will be able to stretch farther with greater ease.

4

Bend your torso to the other side and bounce 4 times.

STOMACH

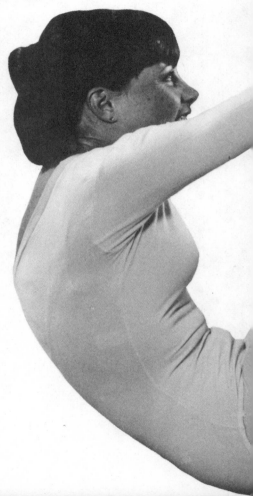

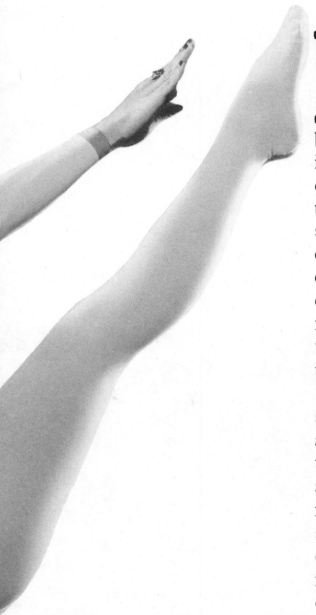

Nothing can do more to ruin the lines of an otherwise good figure than a bulging stomach; fortunately, it's one of the faults that's easiest to control. Two factors usually contribute to a large stomach: overweight and out-of-shape muscles. Sensible eating can help rid you of the excess pounds, and spot reducing can strengthen those underused muscles and flatten unwanted curves.

The muscles that affect the shape of your stomach are the abdominals, the obliques, and the transversalis. When these are in shape, they act as a natural girdle, creating three strong bands of tissue from diaphragm to pelvis. Since they respond quickly to exercise, often showing improvement within a week or two, you'll find that before long your silhouette will be slimmer.

There are two additional benefits to be gained from exercising your stomach muscles. Their purpose is to hold the organs of your abdominal cavity in place, and when properly toned they perform this function with optimum efficiency. Also, exercises for the stomach tend to strengthen the muscles of your lower back, easing back pain and improving posture.

Some of the spot reducing exercises that follow are rather strenuous. Give yourself a good workout, but don't overdo. The rapid improvement you'll experience will soon enable you to increase the difficult movements, and in no time at all you'll have a flat, strong stomach.

CLASSIC SIT-UP

If you can't do the complete sit-up, start in a sitting position and lower your body to the count of four. Whether you do half or complete sit-ups, keep your stomach pulled in and your back rounded throughout the sequence.

To Reduce: complete 4 sit-ups or 8 half sit-ups

Maintenance: add 4 sit-ups per week, working up to 16 to 24

1

Lie flat on your back with knees bent and feet flat on the floor. Clasp your hands behind your neck.

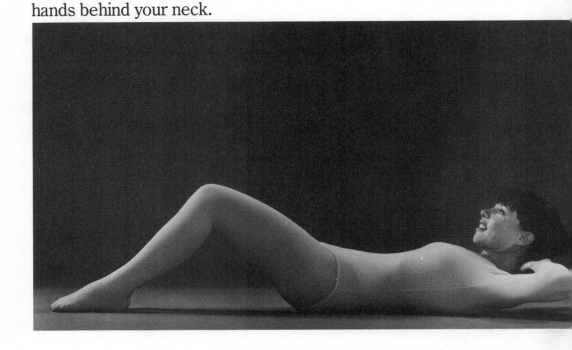

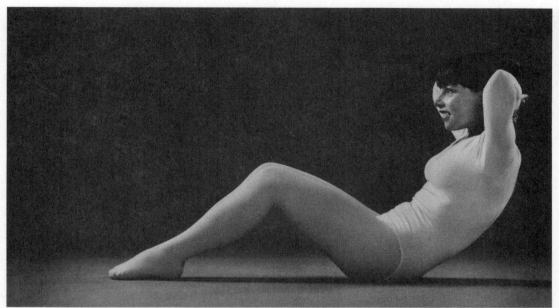

2

Slowly bring your torso up into a sitting position, with your back rounded. Keep your feet flat on the floor.

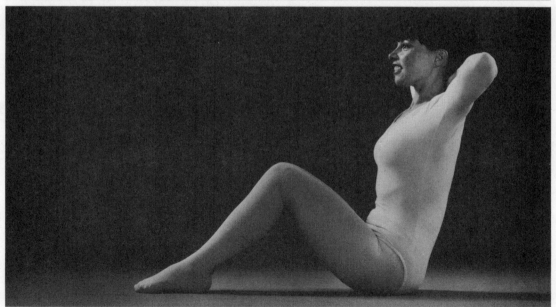

3

When you reach a sitting position, straighten your back, keeping your stomach pulled in. Hold. Round your back and lower your torso slowly to the floor.

ANKLE CATCH

This exercise looks easy, but you may find it difficult at first to clasp your ankle. If so, take hold of your calf for that part of the sequence until you're able to reach farther.

To Reduce: repeat sequence 4 times, alternating legs

Maintenance: repeat sequence 12 times, alternating legs

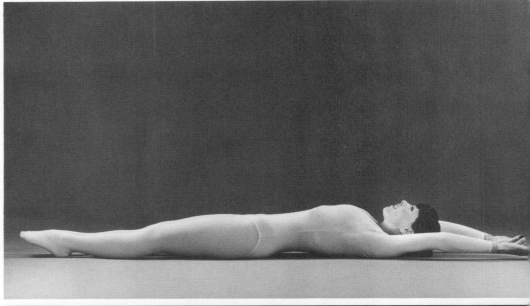

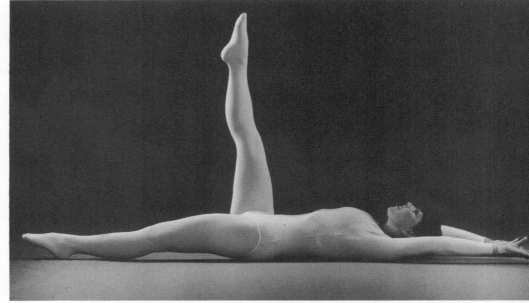

1

Lie on your
back, legs
straight and feet
pointed, with
your arms
stretched out on
the floor behind
your head.

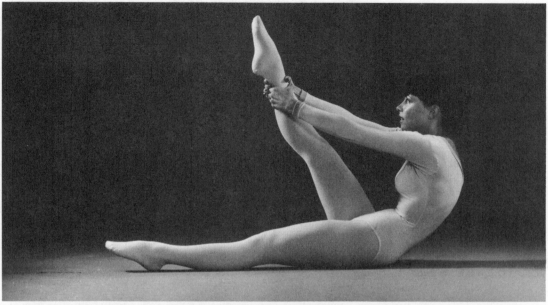

3

Swing your arms
up, raising your
torso into a
sitting position.
At the same
time, keeping
your back
rounded, clasp
the ankle of your
right leg with
both hands.

2

Raise your right
leg until it is
perpendicular to
the floor. Keep
both legs
straight and feet
pointed.

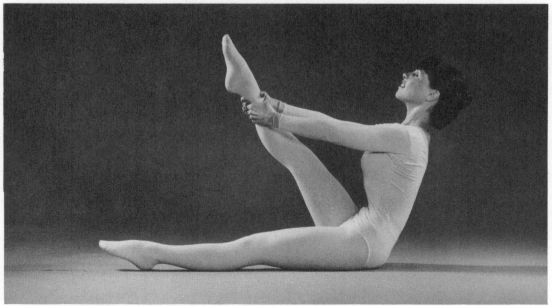

4

Without bending
your right knee,
straighten your
back and pull in
your stomach.
Hold for 3
seconds. Return
to the original
position. Repeat
with left leg.

AIR CYCLING

"Bicycling" in the air is a standard and effective exercise for flattening the tummy. If it causes any back pain, however, consult your doctor before continuing.

To Reduce: repeat sequence 4 times

Maintenance: repeat sequence 8 times

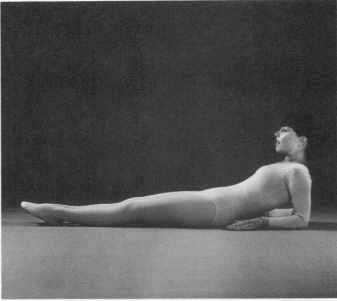

1

Lie on the floor with your torso propped up on your elbows. Your legs should be straight, feet together and pointed, and your forearms should be parallel to your body. Keep the palms of your hands flat on the floor.

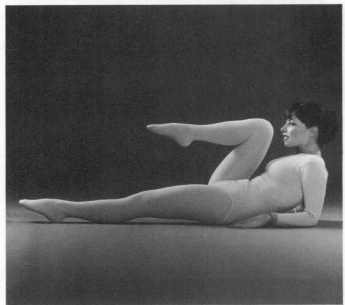

2

Bend your right knee and bring it up to your chest.

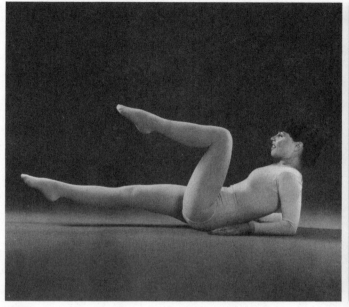

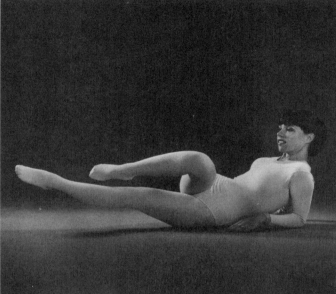

4

Lean onto the left side of your fanny and pedal 8 times with each leg; then lean onto the right side and pedal 8 more times with each leg.

3

As you straighten the knee and lower your right leg to within 6 inches of the floor, bend your left knee and bring it up to your chest. When you straighten your left leg, lower it to within 6 inches of the floor while you bend your right knee to your chest. The alternating movement should resemble pedaling a bicycle. Keep your stomach muscles tightened. Make 8 pedaling motions with each leg.

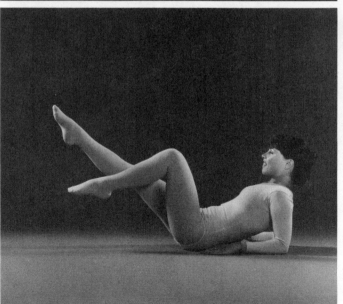

5

Return to the original position and make the cycling motions 8 final times with each leg.

THE BODY FOLDS

Excellent for trimming the tummy, this exercise may have to be limited to one sequence when you begin. As your stomach muscles become stronger, however, it becomes less difficult.

To Reduce: repeat 4 times

Maintenance: add 4 times a week, working up to 20

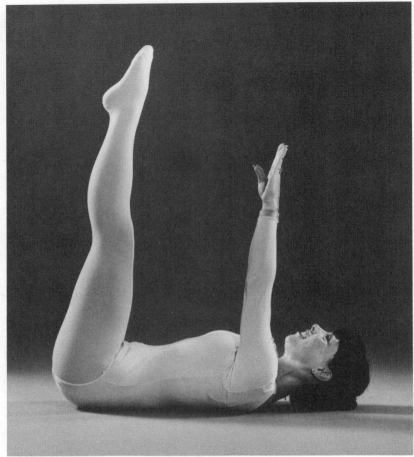

1

Lie flat on your back with your arms and legs stretched straight up in the air so that your body forms a U. Your feet should be pointed.

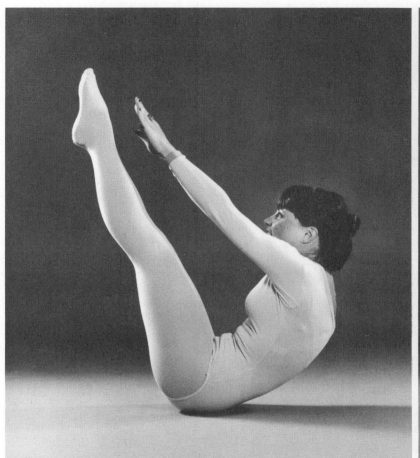

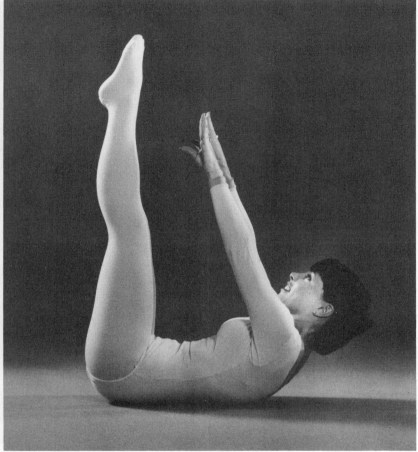

2

Keeping your stomach
pulled in, lift your back
and torso off the floor and
reach for your feet, all in
one movement.

3

Relax to the original
position, being sure to
keep your arms and legs
perpendicular to the
floor.

STOMACH

UP, UP AND AROUND

This exercise is strenuous, but it produces results quickly. If any back pain occurs, consult your doctor. You may find that altering the exercise slightly by making small arcs with your legs and keeping them higher off the floor will eliminate the pain. After several weeks, you should be able to do the exercise as described. Keep your feet pointed throughout.

To Reduce: repeat sequence 4 times from step 2

Maintenance: add 4 times a week, working up to 12

58

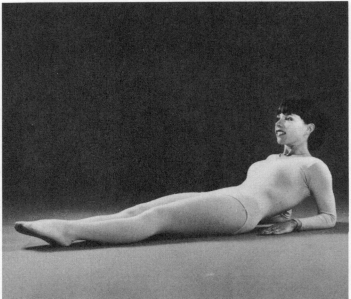

1

Lie on the floor with your torso propped up on your elbows. Your legs should be straight, feet together and pointed, and your forearms should be parallel to your body. Keep your palms flat on the floor.

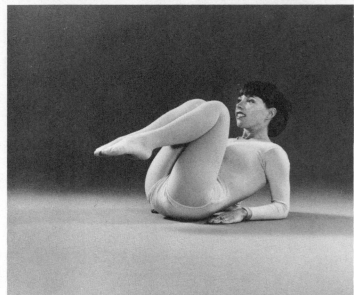

2

Bend both knees, bringing them up to your chest. Make sure your stomach muscles are tightened.

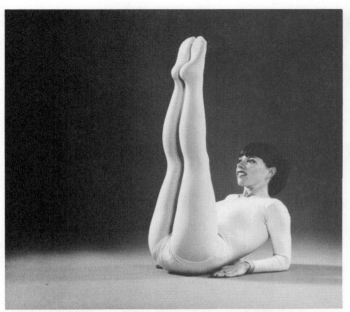

3

Straighten both legs so they are perpendicular to the floor. Do not rock back on your shoulders.

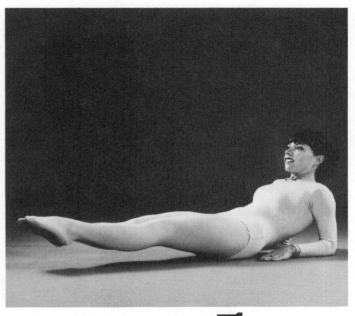

4

Separate your legs. Making wide arcs with each leg, begin to lower them slowly without bending your knees.

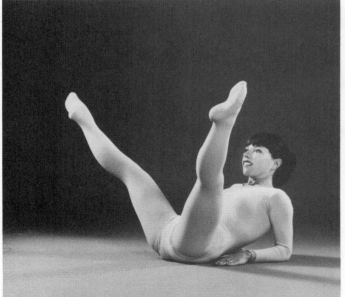

5

When your legs are about 10 inches from the floor, bring them together. Hold this position for 2 seconds, keeping your stomach muscles tightened. Bring your knees up to your chest, as in step 2, and repeat.

STAR GAZING

In this exercise, you lower your back only slightly. It is important to contract your stomach muscles as you raise and lower your back.

To Reduce: repeat 8 times

Maintenance: repeat 16 times

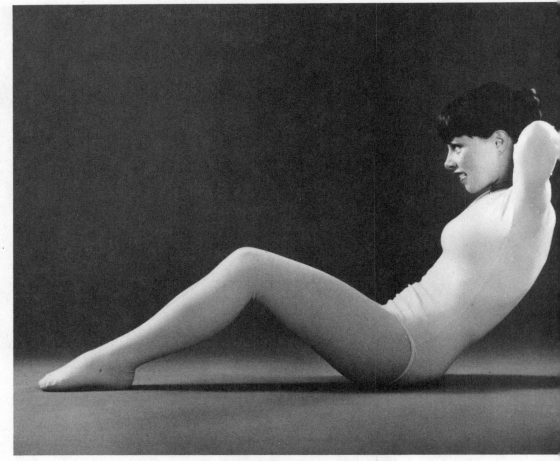

1

Sit with your knees bent, touching, and your feet flat on the floor. Clasp your hands behind your neck with your elbows straight out to the side. Contract your stomach and slowly round your back as you lower it slightly toward the floor.

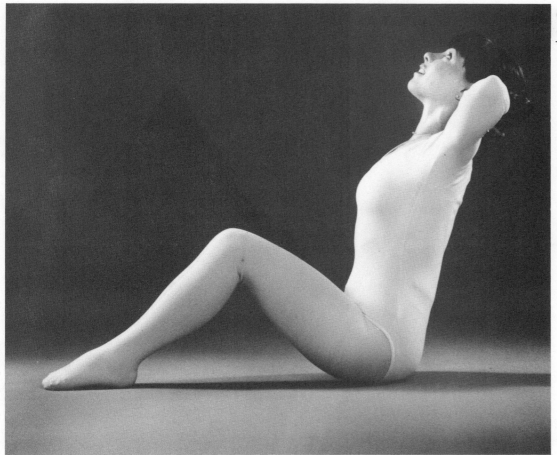

2

Keeping your stomach contracted, sit up straight while lifting your face to look up at the ceiling. Keep your knees bent and your feet on the floor. Hold this position for 2 seconds, then round your back slightly and relax your stomach.

BASIC BELLY DANCER

By contracting and releasing your stomach muscles, you can trim your stomach and strengthen your lower back. This is an especially good exercise to do to music.

To Reduce: repeat 16 times

Maintenance: as often as you wish, but at least 16 times

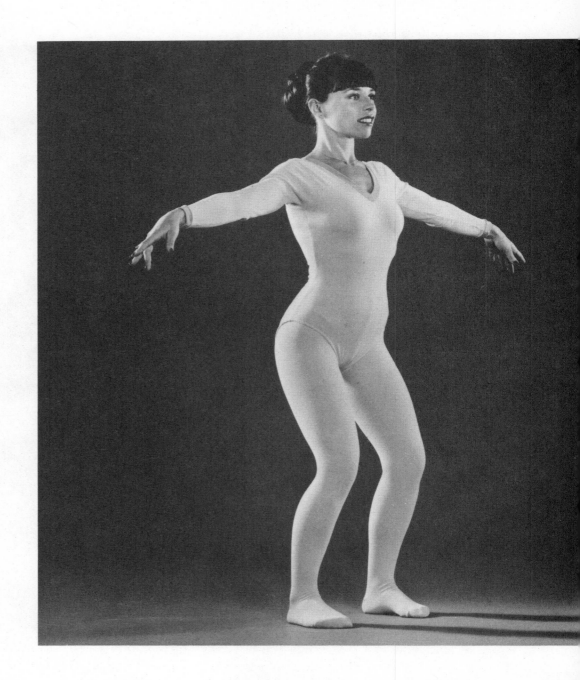

1

Stand with your feet parallel and about 8 inches apart, knees slightly bent and arms relaxed at shoulder level. Tighten your stomach and stick out your fanny, arching your lower back.

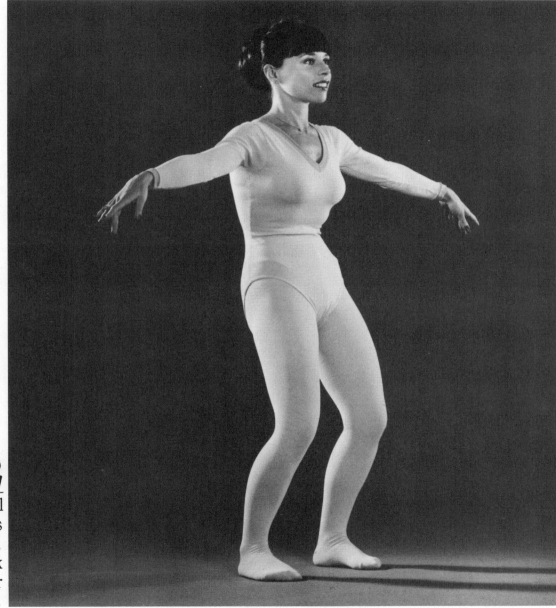

2

With your knees still bent, tuck your pelvis under as far as you can, rounding your lower back and contracting your stomach muscles.

WAIST & MIDRIFF

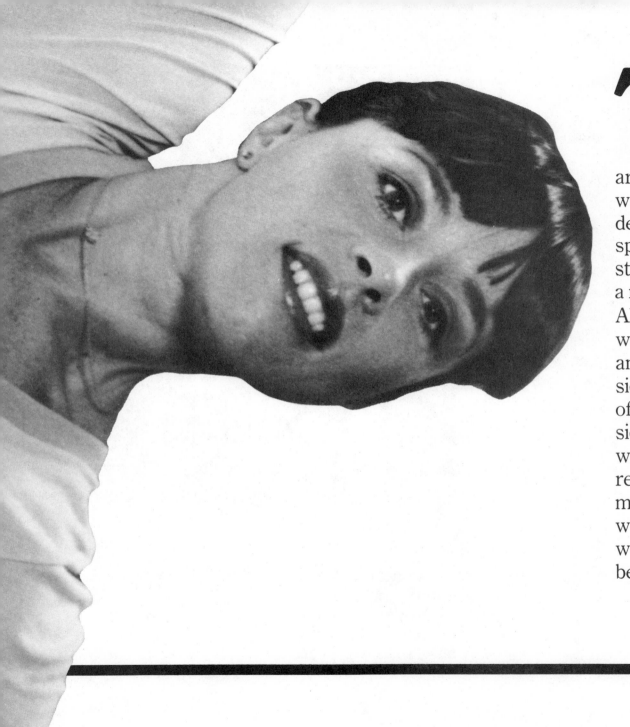

The days of the hourglass figure and tightly corseted middle are long gone; but a narrow waist is still attractive and desirable. Combining spot reducing exercises for stomach and waist will produce a narrow, flat midsection. All the exercises in this section work to trim the serratus anterior muscles, located on the sides of your torso. And some of them strengthen both the sides and the front of your waist. Many of these exercise require twisting and stretching movements. After only a few weeks, you should feel your waist and entire midriff becoming tighter and firmer.

PELICAN TWIST

To prevent dizziness, look at the floor while you twist your torso. Do not exceed 16 twists, or you may strain your muscles.

To Reduce: repeat sequence 8 times

Maintenance: repeat sequence 16 times

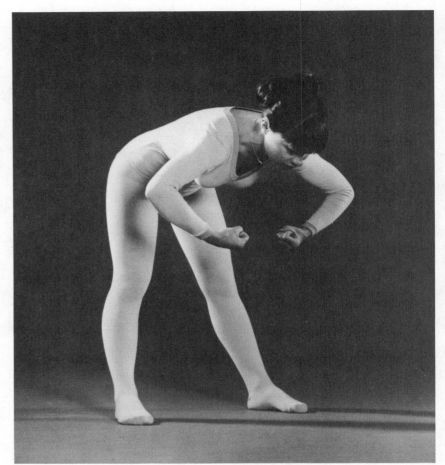

1

Stand straight with your feet apart. Bend forward at the hips but keep your back straight. Make your hands into fists and bend your arms with the elbows sticking out to the side. Your fists should almost meet in front of your chest.

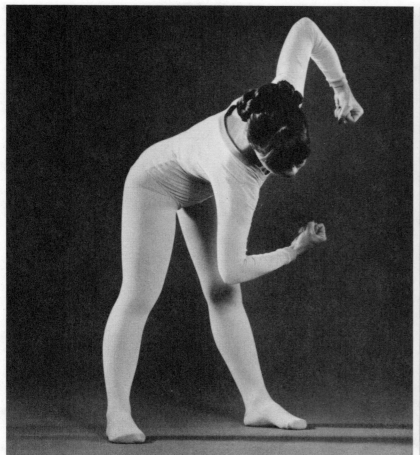

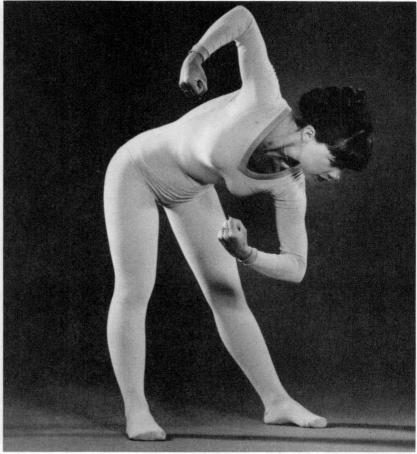

2

Twist your torso up to the
left, keeping your arms in
their original position.
Your left elbow should point
toward the ceiling and your
right elbow toward the floor.

3

Reverse the position of
your body, twisting your
torso up to the right and
raising your right elbow.

ELASTIC "C"

When you do this exercise correctly, you can feel the muscles stretch along your waist and ribs. Do not lean forward or arch your back; be careful to bend directly sideways.

To Reduce: repeat sequence twice

Maintenance: repeat sequence 3 times

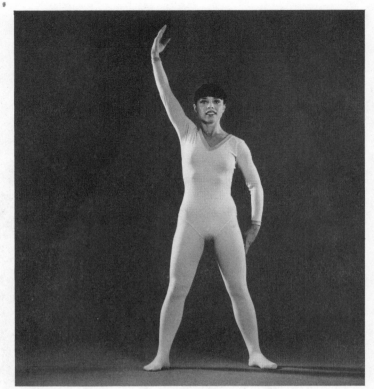

1

Stand straight with your feet apart and stretch your right arm over your head, leaving your left arm relaxed at your side.

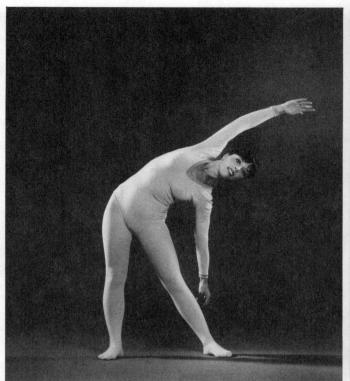

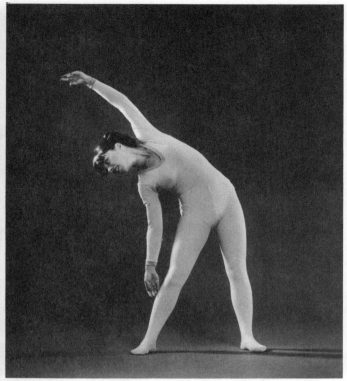

2

Curve your torso to the left without bending forward or arching your back. Reach as far to the left as you can with your right arm. Bounce to the left 8 times, stretching your right arm as far as possible. Keep your left arm relaxed at your side.

3

Reverse arms and bounce 8 times to the right.

ROTATING "C"

Once you get used to the sequence of movements, you'll be able to do this exercise smoothly. Be sure to make a full circular motion with your upper body, stretching from the waist.

To Reduce: repeat sequence 4 times

Maintenance: repeat sequence 8 times

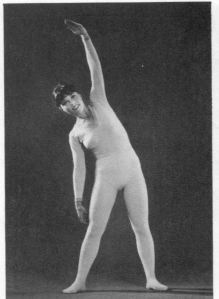

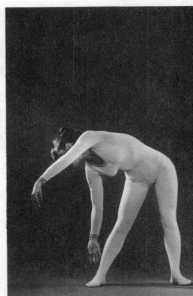

1

Stand straight with your feet apart. Stretch your left arm over your head, leaving your right arm relaxed at your side.

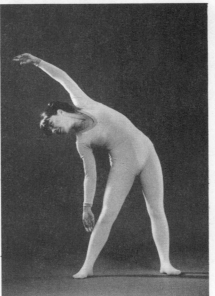

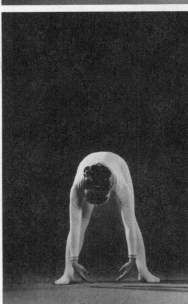

2

Curve your torso to the right without bending forward or arching your back. Reach as far to the right as you can with your left arm. Bounce 4 times to the right.

3

Pause. Twist
your torso so
your chest faces
the floor. Bring
your left hand
down to meet
your right.

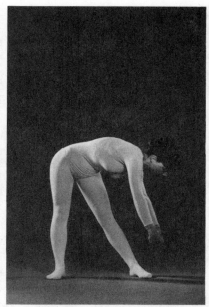

5

Continue the
motion of your
body until your
arms are parallel
to your left leg.
Straighten your
torso and lift
your left arm.

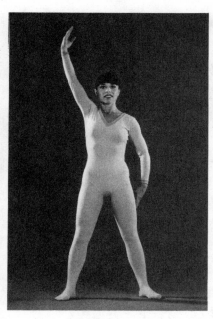

7

Repeat in
reverse, so you
end up in the
original position.

4

Swing your
lowered torso
around so your
arms reach down
in front of you.

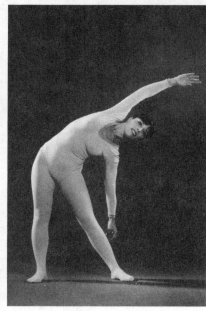

6

As in step 2,
curve your body
and reach to the
left with your
right arm.
Bounce 4 times
to the left.

DOWEL TWIST

You may not be able to keep your arms perfectly straight until after a few weeks of doing this exercise. Bend your arms only when you cannot lower them farther in the straight position. Keep your back straight, not arched, and your stomach muscles tightened. (You may use a broomstick in place of a dowel, but be sure your hands are 3 feet apart.)

To Reduce: complete sequence once

Maintenance: the same

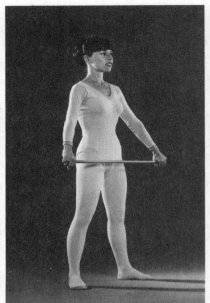
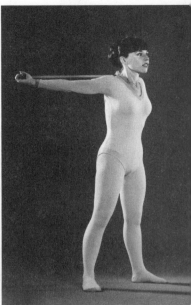

1

Stand with your feet apart and your legs straight, holding a 3-foot dowel (¾ inch in diameter) in front of you with both hands, just below your hips.

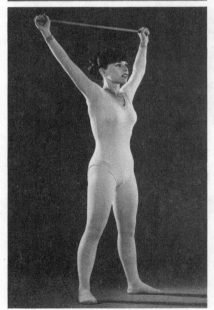
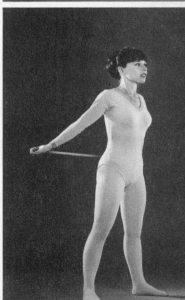

2

Without bending your arms, raise the dowel up over your head.

3

Lower the dowel behind you, keeping your arms as straight as possible. You may have to bend your arms when you first do this exercise, but be sure to maintain the position of your hands.

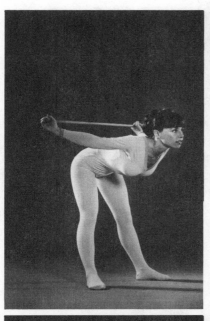

4

Lower the dowel to about 6 inches behind your fanny. Your arms should be straight.

5

Bend forward at the hips without rounding your back, and raise your arms slightly behind you.

6

Twist your torso to the right, lowering your right shoulder and arm. Keep your back straight.

7

Twist your torso to the left, lowering your left shoulder and arm. Twist 8 times in each direction.

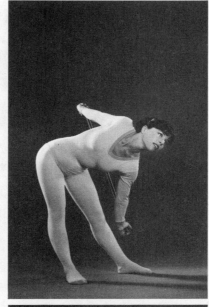

8

Stand up straight and bring the dowel back to its original position in front of you. Again, bend your arms only if you must.

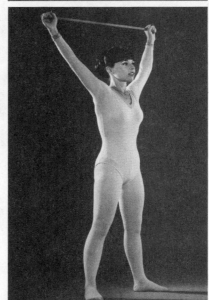

73

COPTER TWIST

When you tighten your stomach and fanny muscles, you'll find it easier to keep your lower body still while your waist and upper body twist. For best results, twist as far as you can to each side.

To Reduce: repeat sequence 8 times

Maintenance: repeat sequence 16 times

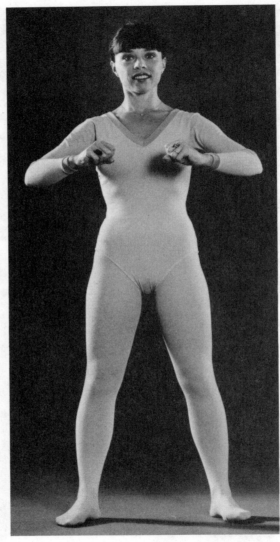

1

Stand straight with your feet apart and your arms bent at chest level, with your upper arms raised slightly away from the body. Make your hands into fists.

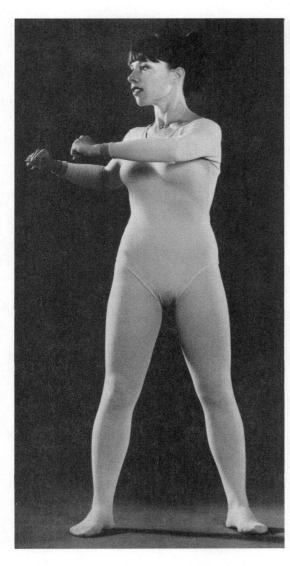

2

Without moving your hips or lower body, twist your torso twice to the right as far as you can.

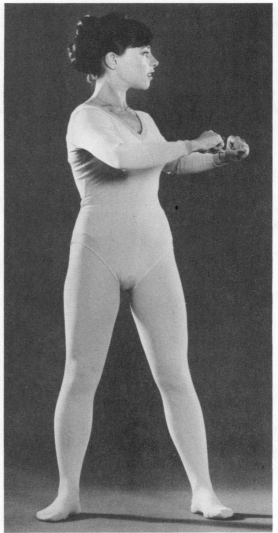

3

In the same manner, twist your torso twice to the left as far as you can.

75

"T" BODY AND TORSO SLIDE

It's a good idea to watch yourself in a mirror as you do this exercise; it isn't effective unless your lower body is completely still.

To Reduce: repeat sequence 12 times

Maintenance: repeat sequence 24 times

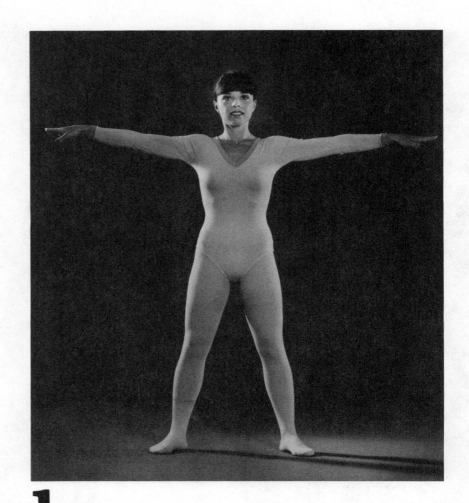

1

Stand straight with your feet apart and your arms stretched out to the side at shoulder height.

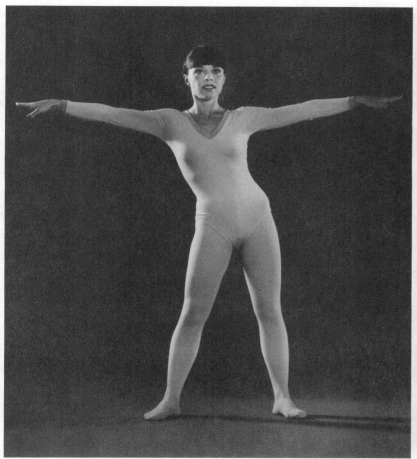

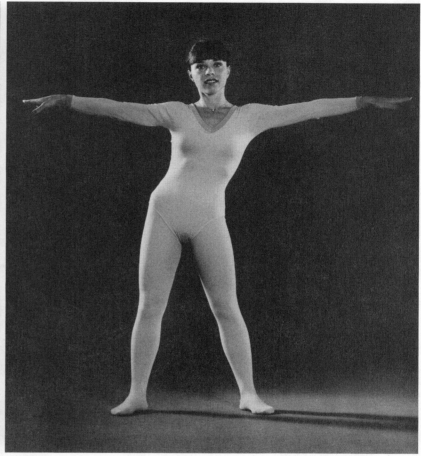

2

Without moving your hips, slide your torso to the right as far as it will go. Keep your shoulders level and your arms straight.

3

In the same manner, slide your torso to the left.

SWINGING BLADE

Some of the exercises in the section for reducing hips and thighs require lifting your foot from the floor. Although this exercise is similar, its purpose is to trim the waist and your foot may brush the floor as you swing your leg around.

To Reduce: repeat sequence 8 times with each leg

Maintenance: repeat sequence 16 times with each leg

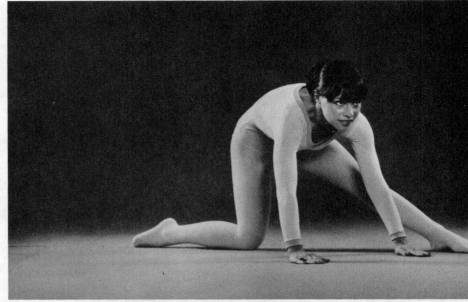

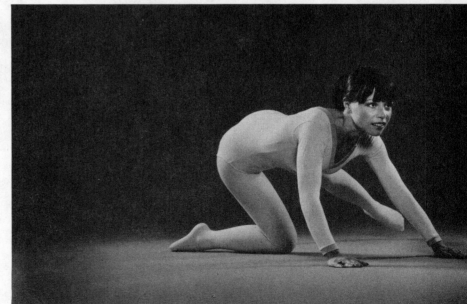

1

Beginning on your hands and knees, straighten your left leg and bring it up next to your left hand with the foot flat on the floor.

2

Swing your left leg out to the side, keeping it absolutely straight. Your foot may brush the floor.

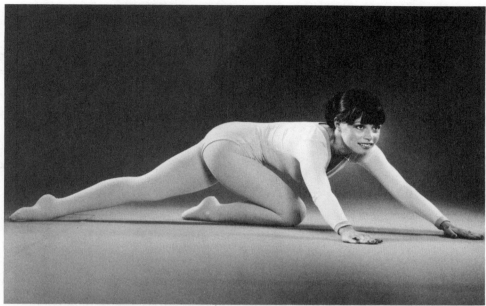

3

Continuing the motion, stretch your leg out behind you and around as far as possible to your right. As your leg swings around, lower your body so you are almost crouching.

4

Swing the foot up to your left hand again, raising your body to the original position and keeping your leg straight.

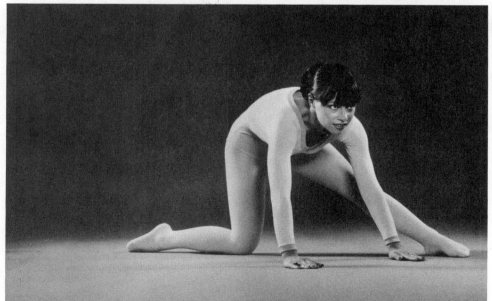

STRETCH AND BOW

The movements in this stretching exercise resemble yoga, and are very relaxing. It is important to keep your fanny flat on the floor and your stomach pulled in while you bounce.

To Reduce: repeat sequence 4 times

Maintenance: repeat sequence 8 times

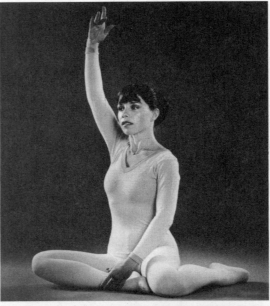

1

Sit with your right leg bent in front of you and your left leg bent to the side. Your right foot should touch your left knee, and your left foot should point backward. Raise your right arm over your head and relax your left arm in front of you.

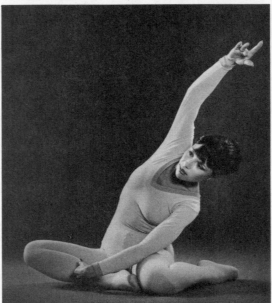

2

Bounce your torso 4 times to the left, stretching your right arm over your head.

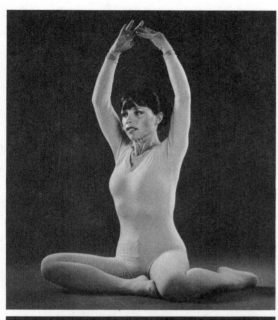

3

Raise your left arm so that your hands meet over your head.

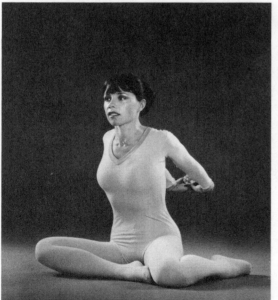

4

Lower your hands behind your back, and clasp them in back of you.

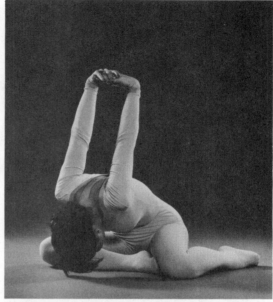

5

Bounce your torso 4 times forward, lifting your arms as high as you can behind you.

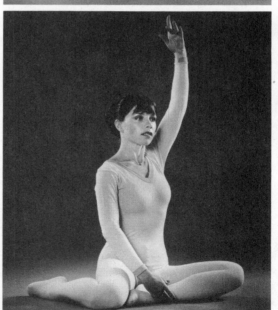

6

Reverse the direction of your legs, raise your left arm, and repeat.

HIPS

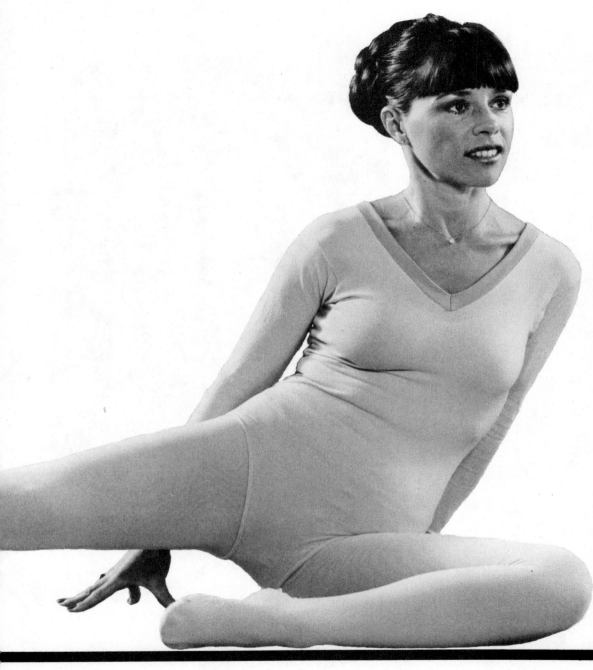

ew women are troubled by heavy hips alone: the problem is usually combined with a spreading fanny, a flabby stomach, or heavy thighs. These are exercises that work specifically to reduce the hip area, getting rid of fat that adds unsightly breadth and bulk.

Exercising the psoas area muscles—the ones that most influence the shape of the hips—will effectively reduce unwanted bulk. Most of the following exercises involve stretches and bends from side to side that will work the psoas. And for double effectiveness, do some of the reducing exercises for the fanny too—many of them work on the psoas as well as the gluteus muscles, which control the fanny.

HIP UP

Keep your stomach and fanny muscles tightened to help you maintain your balance and make this exercise effective.

To Reduce: complete sequence once

Maintenance: complete sequence once, raising and lowering your hip 12 times

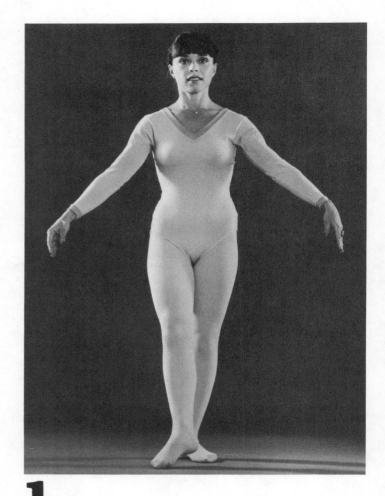

1

Stand with your arms raised away from your body. Bend your right knee slightly and place your weight on your left leg.

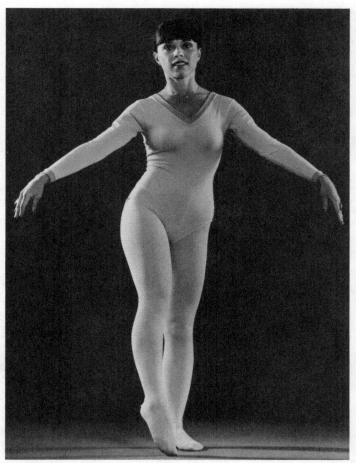

2

Keeping your right knee
slightly bent, raise and
lower your right hip
8 times without lifting
your foot off the floor.

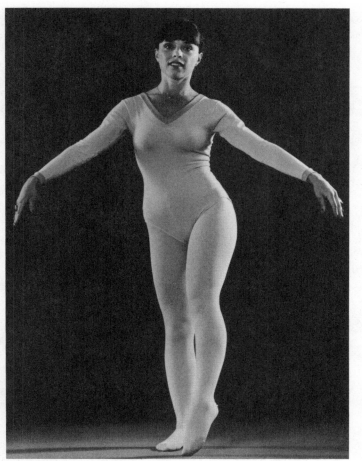

3

Change legs, raising and
lowering your left hip 8
times.

HIP SLIDE

Remember to keep your knees straight and be careful not to arch your lower back.

To Reduce: repeat sequence 8 times

Maintenance: repeat sequence 12 times

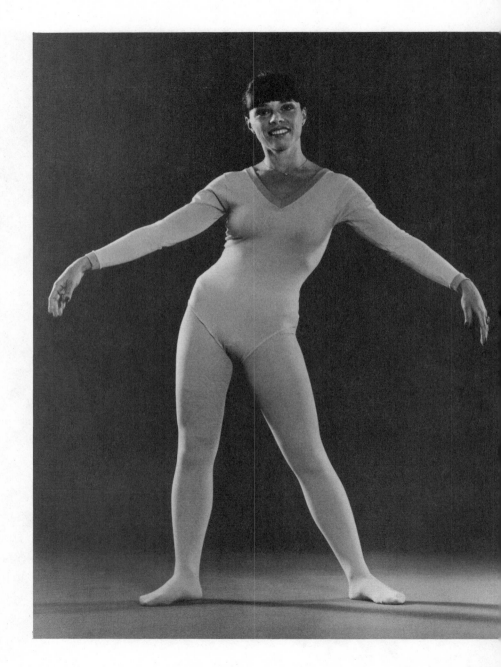

1

Stand with your feet apart and arms raised slightly away from your body. Tighten the muscles in your stomach and fanny. Slide your hips as far to one side as you can, keeping your knees straight and your shoulders as still as possible.

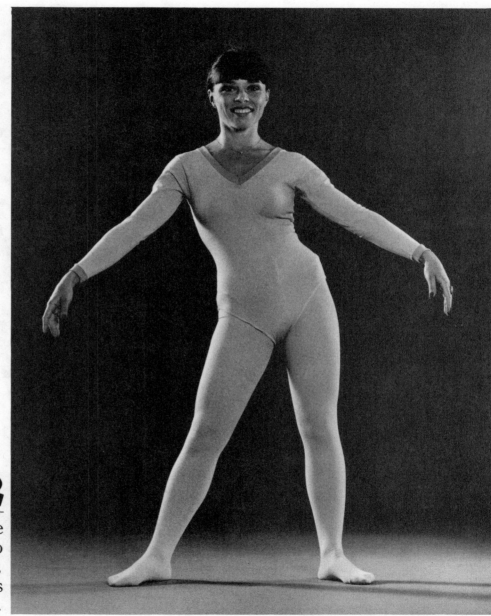

2

Slide your hips to the other side. Be sure not to arch your lower back, and keep your knees straight throughout.

SNAKE HIP CIRCLE

This is another exercise that will bring best results if you keep your stomach and fanny muscles tightened. It is important to remember to lift your hip, not your leg.

To Reduce: complete sequence once

Maintenance: repeat sequence twice

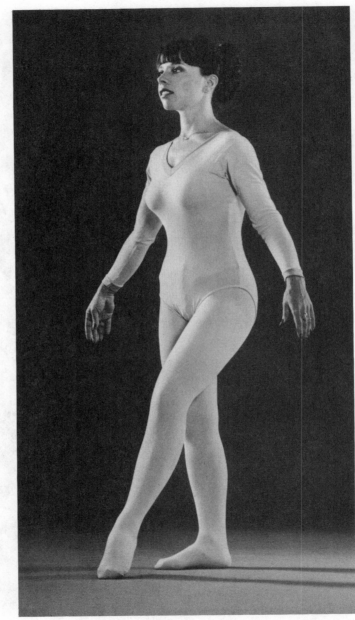

1

Stand with your arms away from your body. Bend your left knee slightly and place your weight on your right leg.

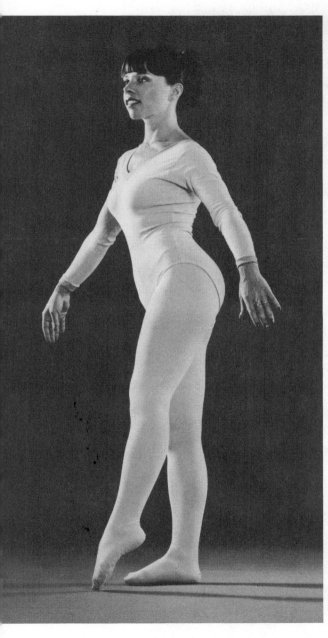

2

Move your left hip in a circle, bringing it forward, up, back, then down. Make 8 circles.

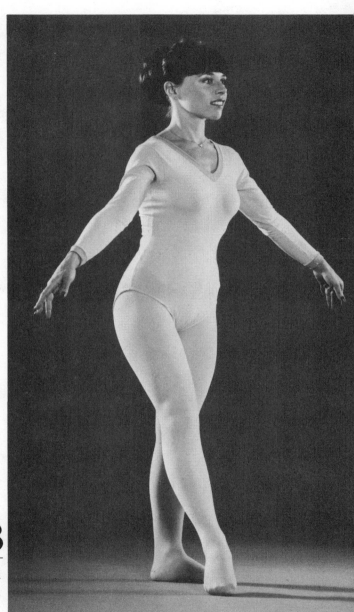

3

Change legs and make 8 circles with the other hip.

DIRECTIONAL SWING

To help maintain your balance during this exercise, hold on to the back of a chair or place the palm of your hand against a wall. Tighten your stomach and fanny muscles and keep both legs straight.

To Reduce: complete sequence once

Maintenance: repeat sequence twice

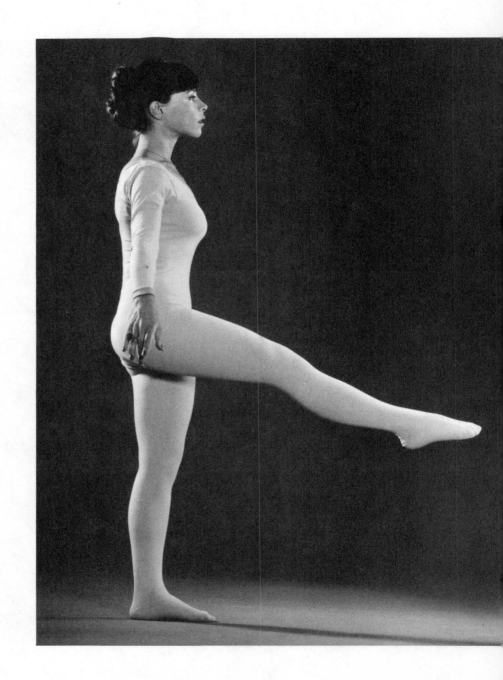

1

Stand with your arms
away from your body and
lift your right leg as high
as you can in front of you.
Keep your knee straight
and foot pointed.

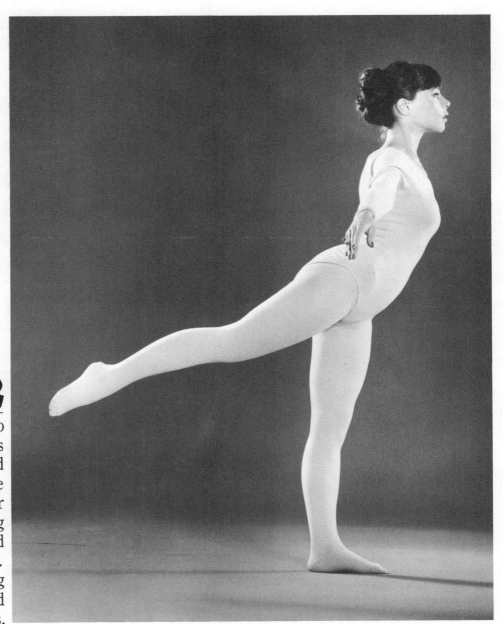

2

Swing your right leg to
the back and raise it as
high as possible behind
you, keeping your knee
straight. Brush the floor
with your foot. Swing
your right leg forward
and back 8 times.
Change sides and swing
your left leg forward and
back 8 times.

PENDULUM SWING

Be sure to keep your knees straight and point the foot of the leg that you swing.

To Reduce: complete sequence once

Maintenance: repeat sequence twice

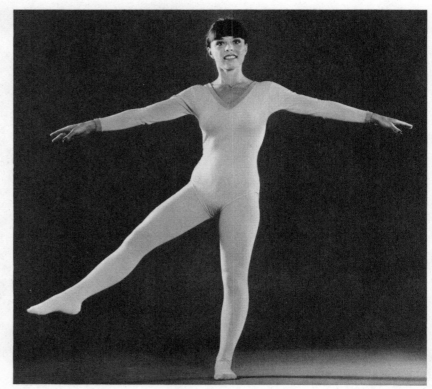

1

Stand with your arms raised almost at shoulder level and lift one leg out to the side. Keep the knee straight and the foot pointed.

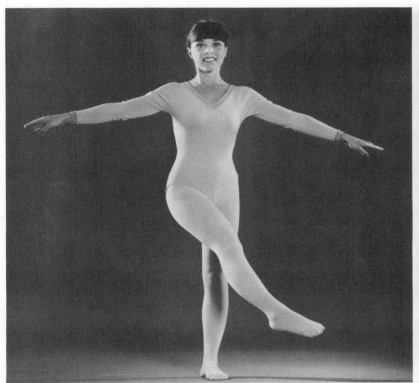 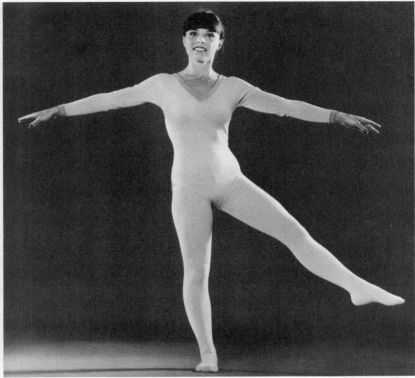

2

Swing the raised leg to the other side, letting your foot brush the floor in front of you. Swing the leg from side to side 8 times.

3

Change sides and swing the other leg 8 times.

"Y" KICK-UP

For best results, do this exercise lying on a hard surface. Lift your leg as high as you can; your hip should leave the floor. Naturally, if you feel strain in your lower back, consult your doctor about the exercise.

To Reduce: complete sequence once

Maintenance: repeat sequence twice

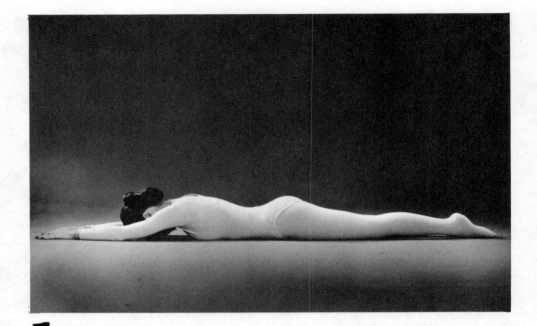

1

Lie on your stomach with your forehead resting on the floor and arms stretched out in front of you. Keep your stomach and fanny muscles tightened.

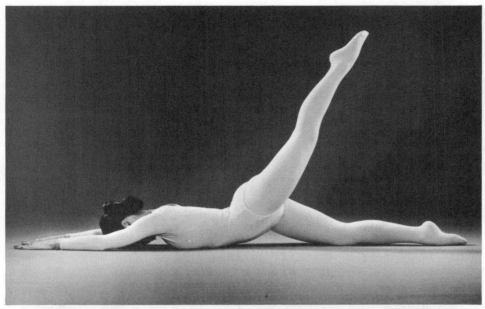

2

Lift your left leg as high off the floor as you can, keeping it straight with the foot pointed. Hold your leg in the air for 2 seconds, then lower it to the floor. Raise and lower your leg 5 times.

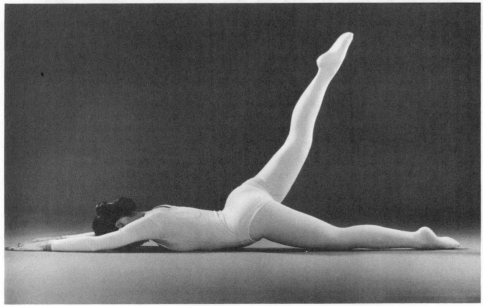

3

Raise and lower your right leg 5 times.

STEM LIFT

Keep your body straight and lift your leg as high as you can. Be sure to stretch your leg, making it as long as possible.

To Reduce: complete sequence once

Maintenance: complete sequence once, raising and lowering your leg 12 times

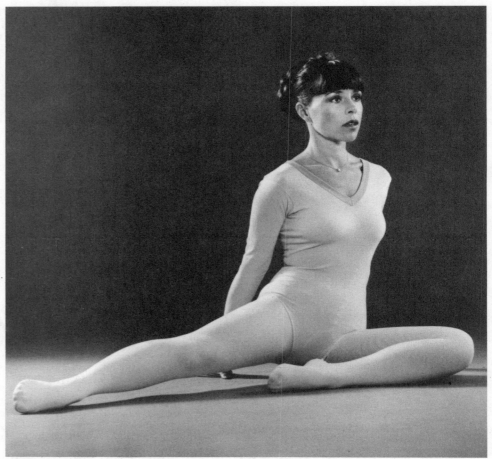

1

Sit with your left leg bent in front of you and your right leg stretched straight out to the side. Place your hands on the floor behind your fanny.

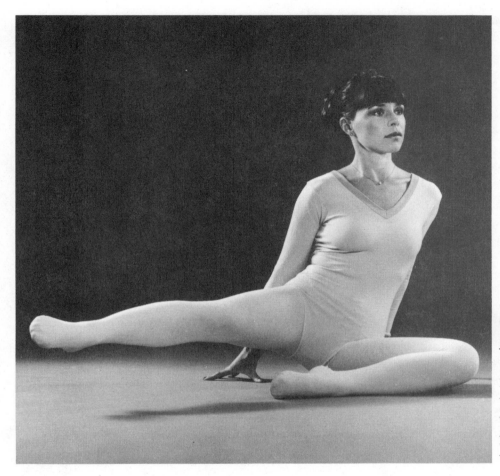

2

Raise and lower your right leg 8 times with your foot pointed and 8 times with your foot flexed. Repeat the series with your left leg.

FANNY

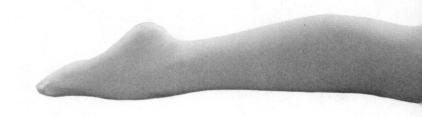

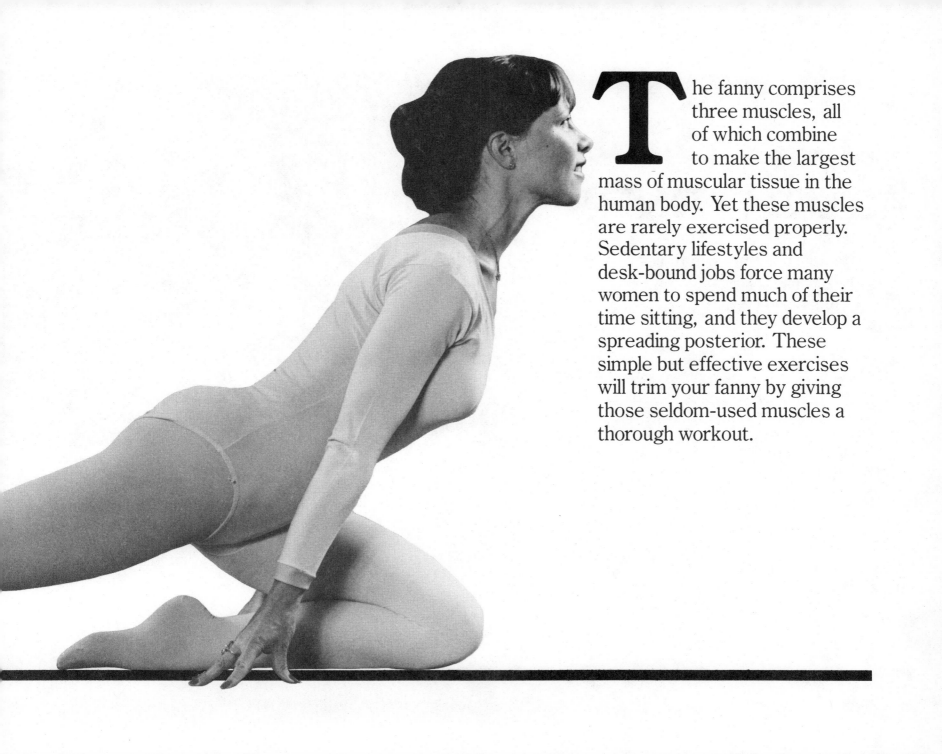

The fanny comprises three muscles, all of which combine to make the largest mass of muscular tissue in the human body. Yet these muscles are rarely exercised properly. Sedentary lifestyles and desk-bound jobs force many women to spend much of their time sitting, and they develop a spreading posterior. These simple but effective exercises will trim your fanny by giving those seldom-used muscles a thorough workout.

THE TIGHTENER

This simple exercise can be done anywhere—standing, sitting, or lying down—and no one will even know you're doing it.

To Reduce: repeat 16 times

Maintenance: repeat 24 times

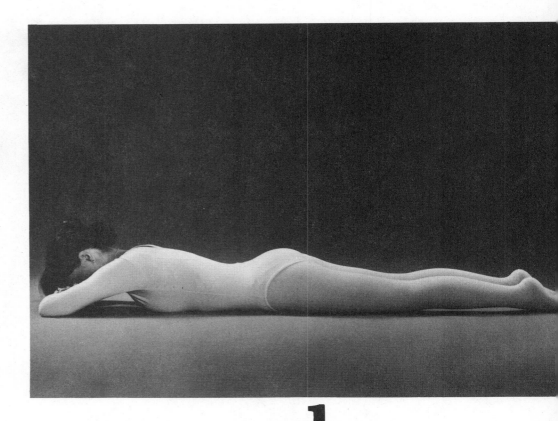

1

Lie on your stomach, resting your forehead on your folded arms. (Or stand or sit tall.)

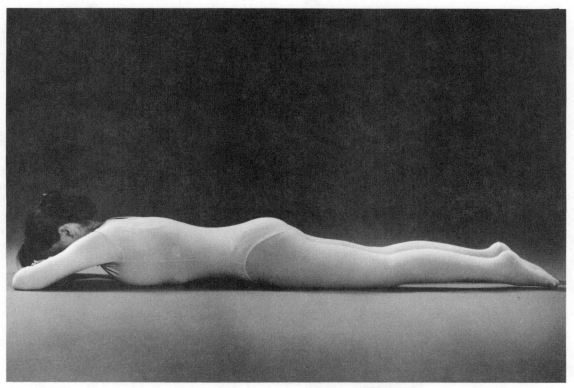

2

Pull in your stomach and
tighten the muscles in
your fanny. Hold this
position for 5 seconds.
Relax.

then to
Bottoms up - page 186

FANNY

STIRRING IT UP

Though it looks easy, this is actually a difficult exercise—but one of the best for tightening and lifting the fanny. Relax and stretch for a moment after completing the exercise.

To Reduce: repeat sequence twice

Maintenance: the same

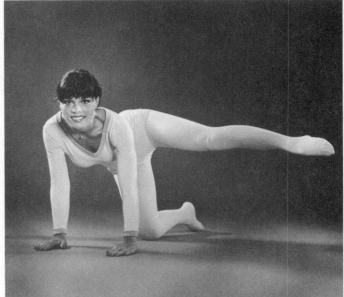

1

Starting on your hands and knees, stretch your left leg out to the side and lift it as high off the floor as comfortably possible. Keep your knee straight and your foot pointed. Your leg should be parallel to the floor.

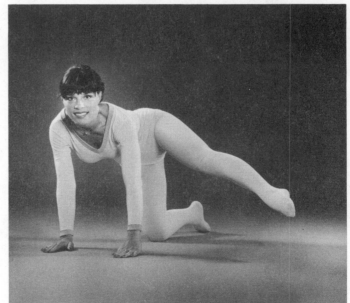

2

Begin a slow rotation of your left leg, moving it forward, then lowering it to within 2 inches of the floor. Keep your knee straight and your body in its original position.

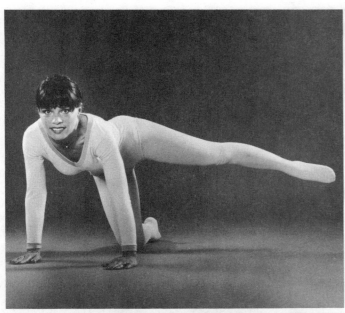

3

Move your leg back, then up, making a full circle.

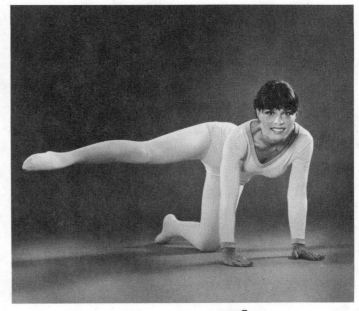

4

Return your leg to the original outstretched position. Make 4 clockwise rotations, then 4 counterclockwise.

5

Repeat the rotations with your right leg.

DONKEY KICK

When you stretch your leg into the air, do not allow your hip to twist upward; keep both hips parallel to the floor.

To Reduce: repeat 8 times with each leg

Maintenance: repeat 12 times with each leg

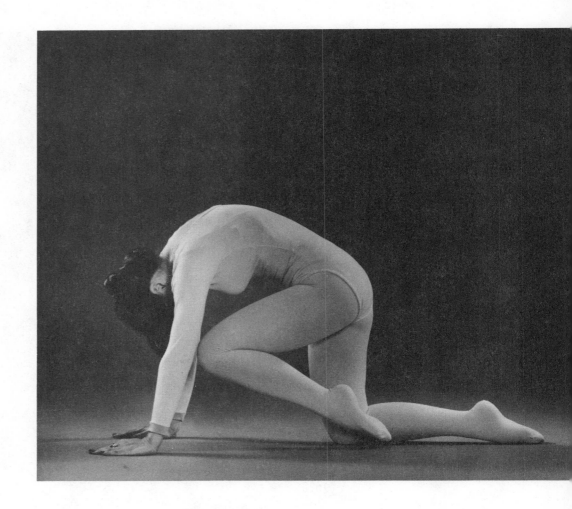

1

Beginning on your hands and knees, lower your head, round your back, and bring one knee in under your body as close to your head as possible. Pull in your stomach and tighten the muscles in your fanny.

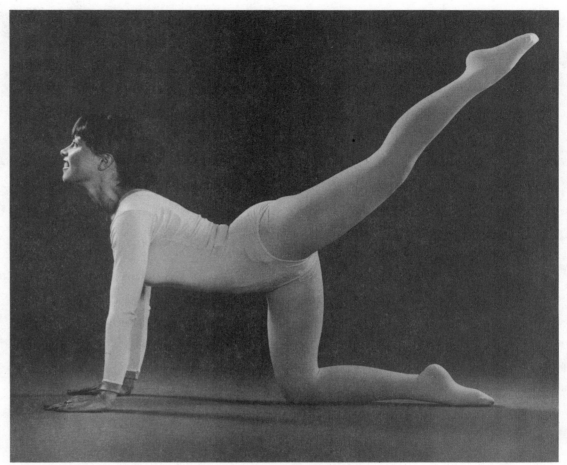

2

In one continuous motion, lift your head and kick your bent leg straight back and up behind you. Your knee should face the floor and the sole of your foot should face the ceiling. Bend your knee and bring you leg back under your body.

WATER PUMP KICK

While you raise and lower your leg, make sure your knee faces forward. Tighten your stomach and fanny muscles throughout. Keep your head up and your back straight.

To Reduce: complete sequence once

Maintenance: the same

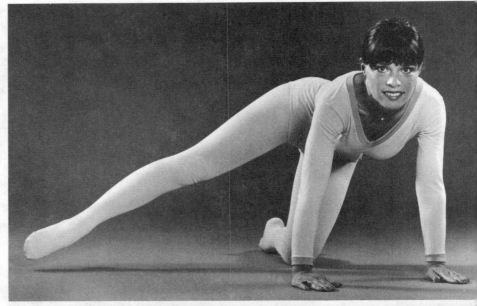

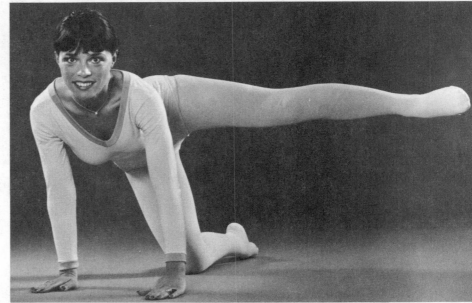

1

Beginning on your hands and knees, stretch your right leg out to the side, with your big toe resting on the floor and knee facing forward. Raise and lower your right leg 16 times. Keep it straight and lift it as far from the floor as you can.

2

Switch sides and raise and lower your left leg 16 times, with the knee straight and the foot pointed.

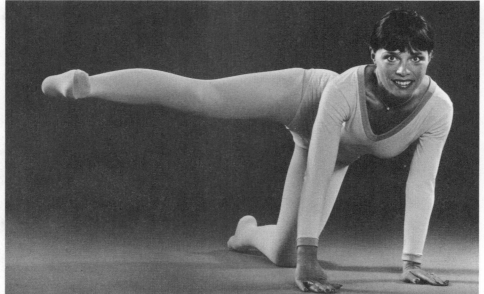

3

Return to the original position, stretching your right leg out to the side but flexing your foot. Raise and lower your right leg 16 times.

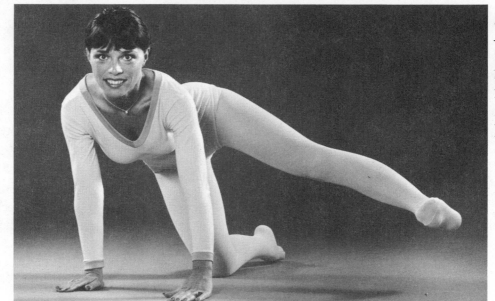

4

Change sides, flex your left foot, and raise and lower your left leg 16 times.

TOE DIPPING

Lowering your feet all the way may prove too difficult at first. Do not force them down; try to lower your legs a little bit more each time you do the exercise, until you're able to touch the floor behind your head with your feet. Keep your feet pointed.

To Reduce: raise and lower your legs 6 times

Maintenance: raise and lower your legs 12 times

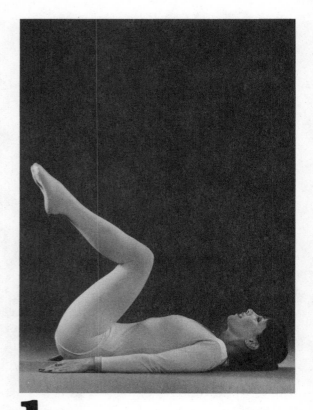

1

Lie on your back with your arms straight at your sides. Bend your knees and bring them up toward your chest.

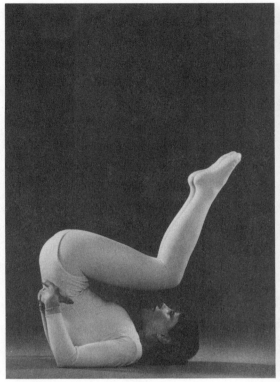

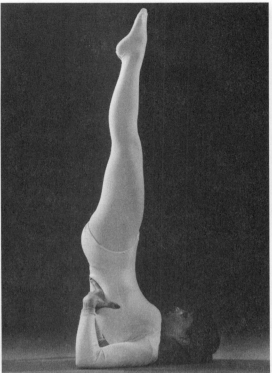

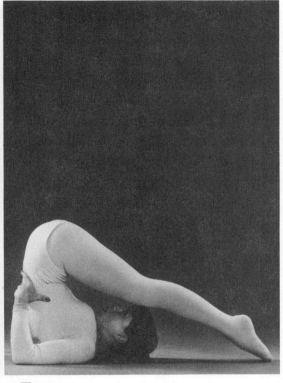

2

Swing your
knees back
toward your
head, bringing
your fanny up off
the floor.
Support your
lower back with
your hands.

3

Raise your legs
straight up in the
air. Your weight
will be on your
shoulders and
your upper arms.
Pull in your stomach
and tighten the
muscles in your
fanny.

4

Slowly lower your
legs backward,
keeping them straight,
until your toes touch
the floor behind your
head. Keeping
your legs straight,
raise them up in
the air and lower
them 6 times.

DOUBLE DONKEY KICK

This exercise is fun to do, but don't get carried away and lose your balance.

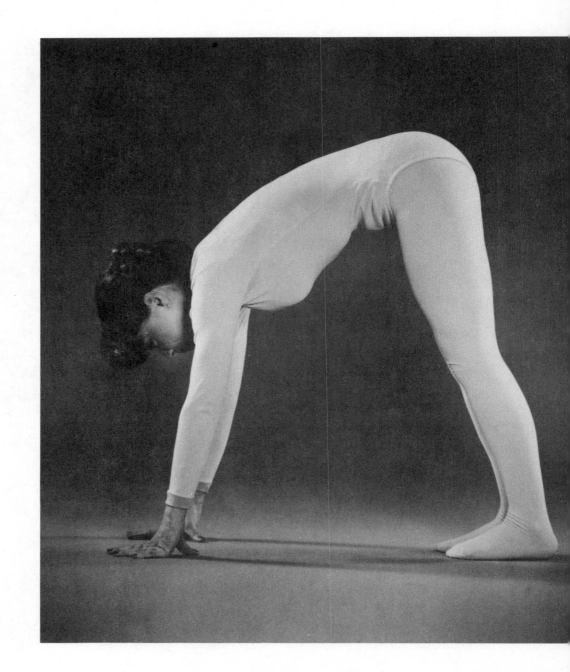

To Reduce: repeat 8 times

Maintenance: repeat 12 times

1

Begin on your hands and feet, with your hands well out in front of your feet and your weight distributed evenly between them.

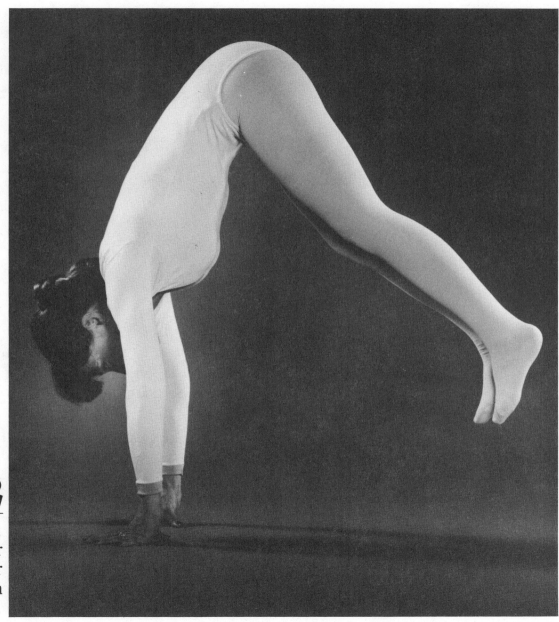

2

Bend your knees slightly, then jump so that your fanny is lifted into the air and all your weight is on your hands.

111

SEESAW TILT

This exercise doesn't look difficult, but you may find it hard to lift your leg far from the floor. After a few weeks, your strength will increase and you'll be able to lift your leg higher.

To Reduce: repeat 4 times on each side, changing sides after 2

Maintenance: repeat 8 times on each side, changing sides after 4

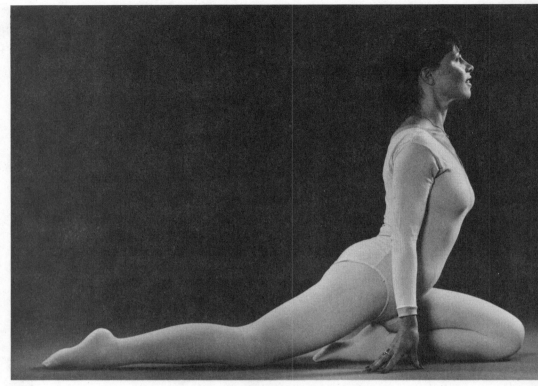

1

Sit on the floor with your left leg bent under you and your right leg stretched out straight behind you. Your left foot and the front of your right leg should be in contact with the floor and pointing straight back. Your arms should be straight at your sides, with fingertips resting on the floor and pointing backward. Pull in your stomach and tighten your fanny muscles.

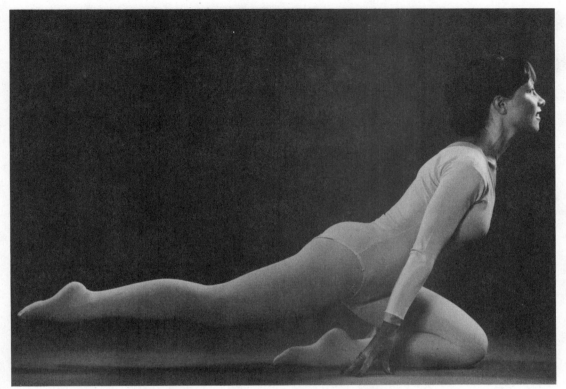

2

Lean forward and raise
your right leg as high as
you can. Be sure to keep
your head raised, knee
straight and foot pointed.

THIGHS

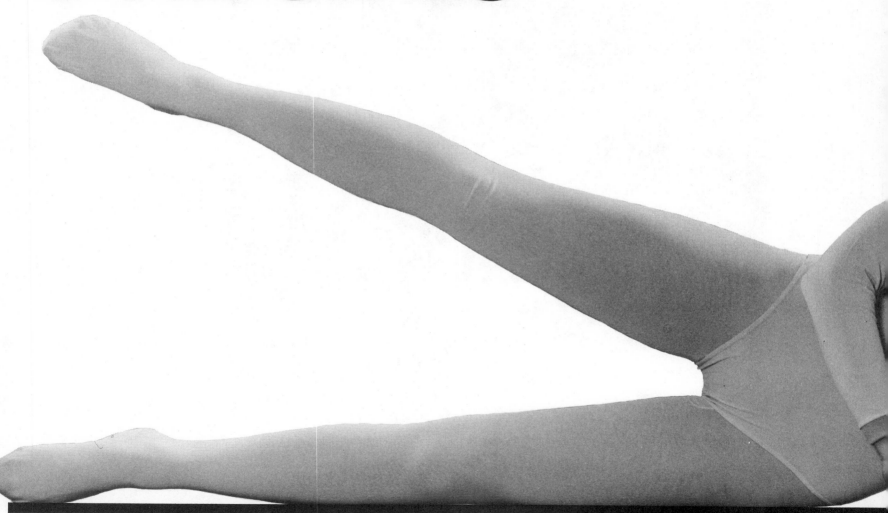

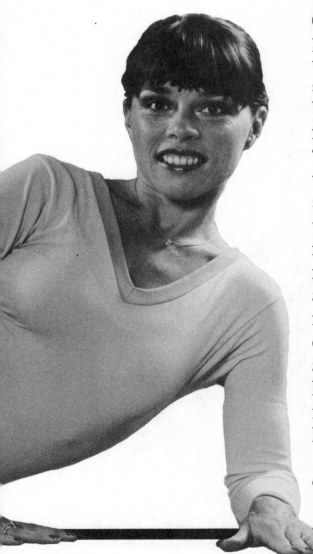

Heavy thighs seem to be the most common and stubborn figure problem for women—even for those who are otherwise satisfied with their bodies. Whether the problem is soft, flabby inner thighs, firm "saddlebags" of fat on the outer thighs, or overall plumpness, spot reducing can help. Most women don't ordinarily perform movements that exercise the muscles at the tops of their legs and keep them firm. The routines that follow were designed to trim those muscles, and will also develop the long, lean muscles that are the foundation of strong, shapely legs.

These exercises affect the quadriceps femoris, located at the front of your thighs, and the hamstrings in the back. They also involve lifts and stretches that will trim your inner and outer thighs. The heaviness of thighs can be difficult to control, and progress may seem dishearteningly slow at first. However, if you do these exercises diligently, you'll notice increased firmness in your inner thighs and improved muscle tone in your outer thighs in as little as three weeks. And before long you'll end up with the trim, slender thighs you've always wanted.

SUPINE AIR KICK

It is important to keep your lower back flat on the floor during this exercise; don't let it arch at all, and keep your feet pointed.

To Reduce: repeat 12 times with each leg

Maintenance: repeat 24 times with each leg, changing legs after 12

1

Lie on your back with your arms stretched straight out to the side. Bend your left leg at the knee, keeping the sole of your left foot flat on the floor.

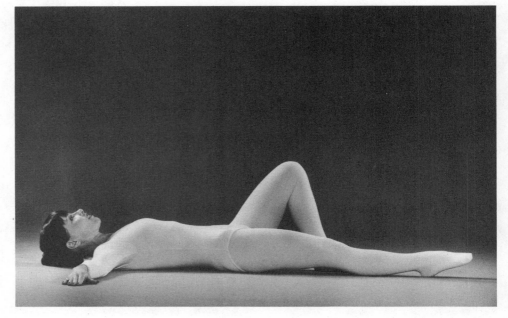

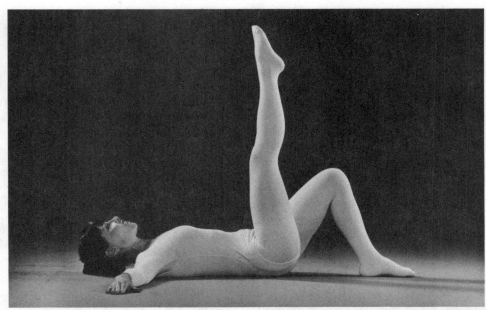

2

Without moving your left leg, lift your right leg until it is perpendicular to the floor. Keep the leg straight and the foot pointed.

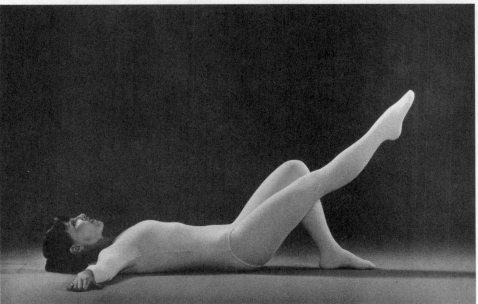

3

Raise and lower your right leg 12 times with the knee straight and the foot pointed.

SUPINE KICK

For maximum effectiveness, bend your knee as tightly as you can and make sure it is completely straight during the kick.

To Reduce: repeat 8 times with each leg, alternating

Maintenance: repeat 12 times with each leg, alternating

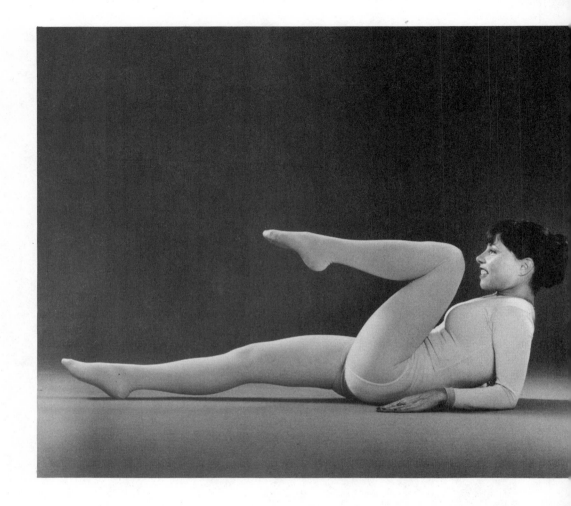

1

Lie on your back, legs straight, feet pointed, and torso propped up on your elbows. Your forearms should be parallel to your body, with the palms of your hands flat on the floor. Bend your left leg and bring the knee up toward your chest.

2

Kick your left leg straight up in the air, perpendicular to your body, and keep your foot pointed. Lower the leg slowly to the floor. Change sides, bending and kicking the other leg.

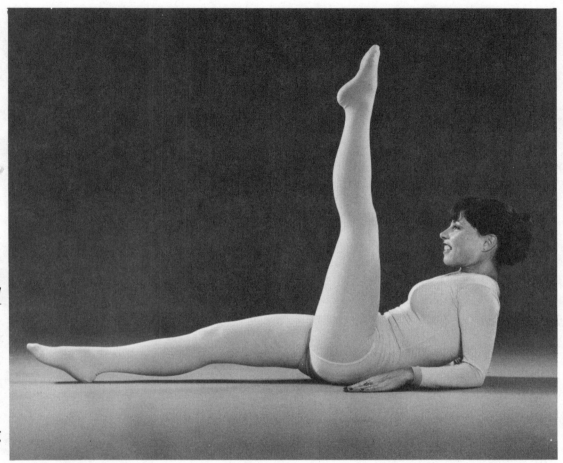

119

PRONE AIR KICK

Don't raise your legs so high
that your hip bones leave the
floor, and make sure your feet
are pointed throughout. If you
feel strain in your lower back,
raise your legs only one or two
inches off the floor to
strengthen lower back muscles.

To Reduce: repeat 16 times
with each leg, alternating

Maintenance: the same

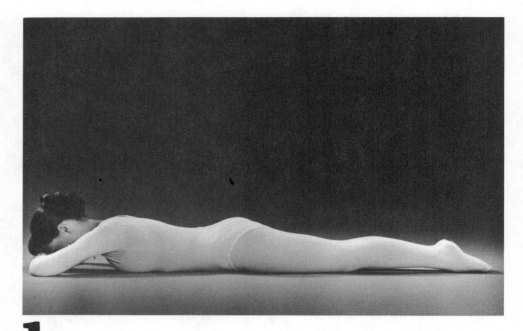

1

Lie on your stomach and
rest your forehead on
your folded arms.

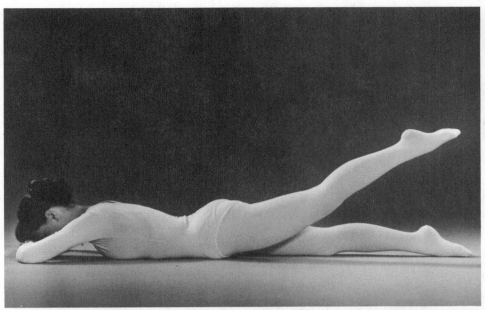

2

Raise your left leg straight into the air with the foot pointed. Hold this position for 2 seconds, then lower your leg to the floor.

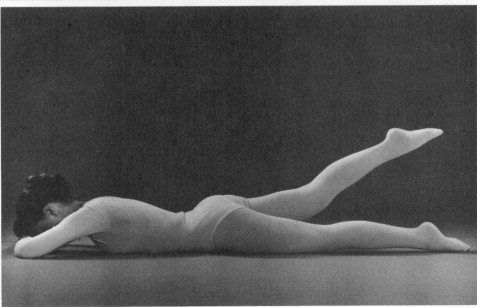

3

In the same manner, raise your right leg, hold the position for 2 seconds, then lower the leg. As you raise your legs, keep your hip bones on the floor and your fanny muscles tightened.

PLIÉ

It's important that you keep your back straight, heels together, and don't allow your fanny to stick out as you bend your knees.

To Reduce: repeat 16 times

Maintenance: repeat 24 times

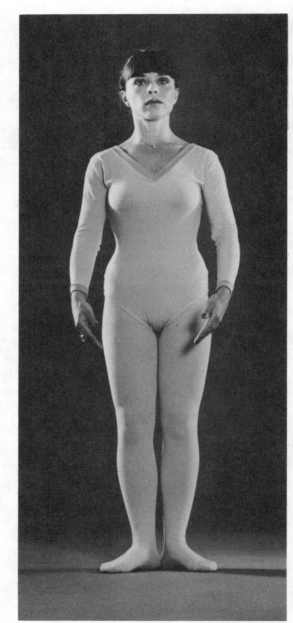

1

Stand straight with your heels together and your toes pointed outward. Your arms should be relaxed at your sides. Keep your stomach pulled in and your fanny muscles tightened.

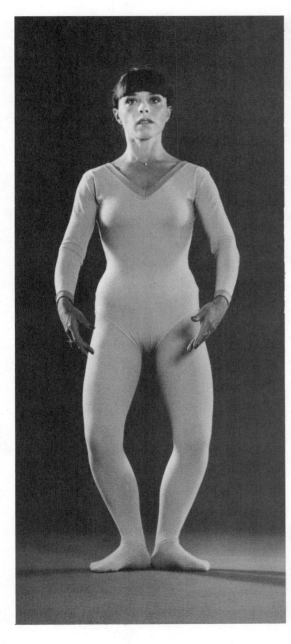

2

Bend your knees and lower your torso about 12 inches. Keep your knees in line with your feet, facing away from your body, and be sure not to arch your lower back.

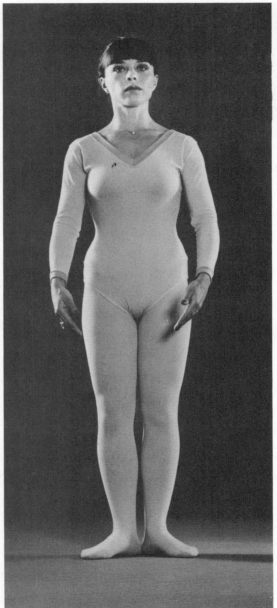

3

Straighten your legs and raise your torso to the original position.

PLIÉ #2

Like the previous exercise, this is a basic ballet movement but requires keeping your feet apart. It increases your flexibility as well as trims your thighs.

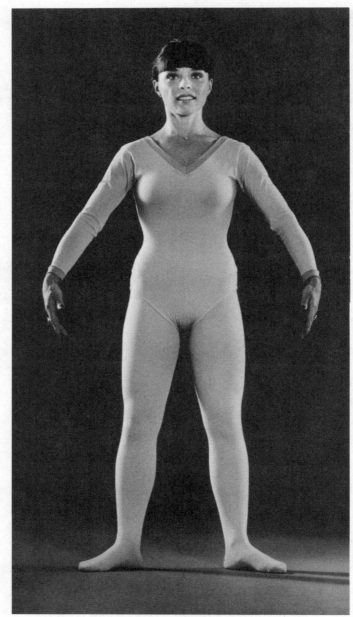

To Reduce: repeat 16 times

Maintenance: repeat 24 times

1

Stand straight with your feet about 6 inches apart and pointed outward. Your arms should be raised slightly away from your body, and your stomach and fanny muscles tightened.

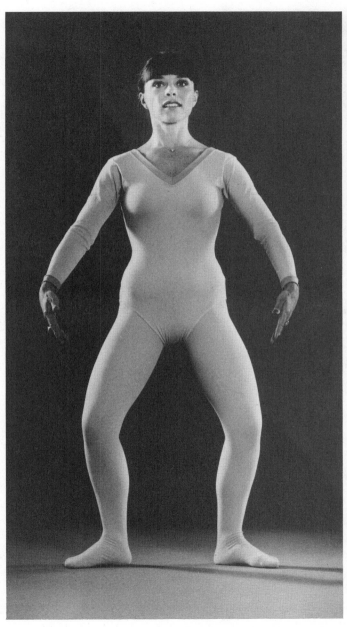

2

Bend your knees and
lower your torso about 12
inches, keeping your
knees in line with your
feet, facing away from
your body. Be sure not to
arch your lower back.
Then, straighten your legs
and raise your torso to
the original position.

GRACEFUL KNEE BEND

In this exercise, it is important to keep your knees facing forward. Tighten your stomach and fanny muscles, but do not tense your shoulders.

To Reduce: repeat 12 times

Maintenance: repeat 24 times

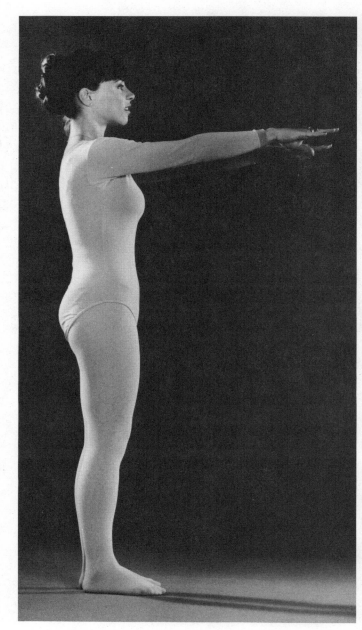

1

Stand straight with your feet slightly apart and parallel, arms stretched straight in front of you at shoulder level.

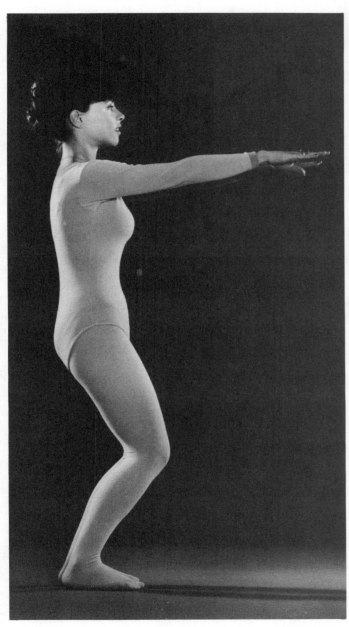

2

Bend your knees slowly
to lower your torso about
12 inches. Keep your
heels flat on the floor and
your back straight.
Slowly straighten your
legs, raising your torso.
Keep your arms out
straight and your knees
facing forward. Be sure
to keep your stomach and
fanny muscles tightened.

ON YOUR MARK

If you do not feel a stretching sensation in the front of your thighs, move the leg you're kneeling on a few inches back.

To Reduce: 16 rocks on each side, changing sides after 8

Maintenance: 18 to 24 rocks on each side, changing sides after 8

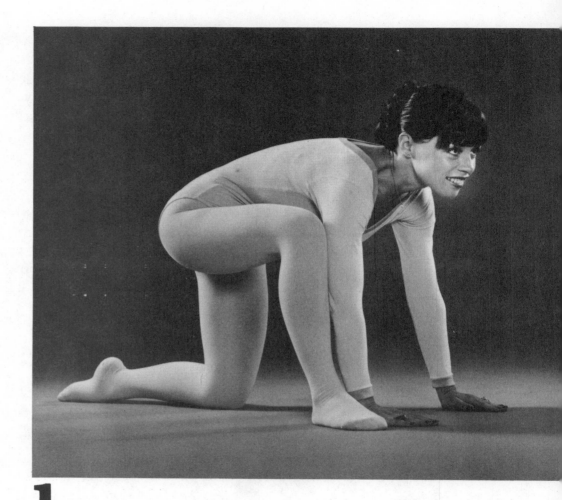

1

Beginning on your hands and left knee, place your right foot next to the outside of your right hand.

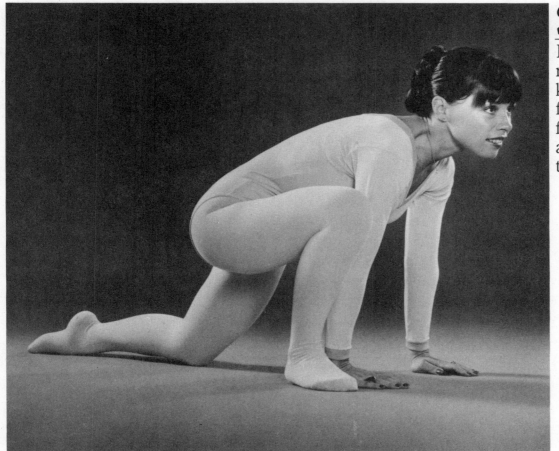

2

Rock forward on your right leg, then back, keeping your heel on the floor and stretching the front of your left thigh and the back of your right thigh.

ON THE BALL

While rocking back and forth, get your body as close as possible to the floor.

To Reduce: 16 rocks, changing sides after 8

Maintenance: the same

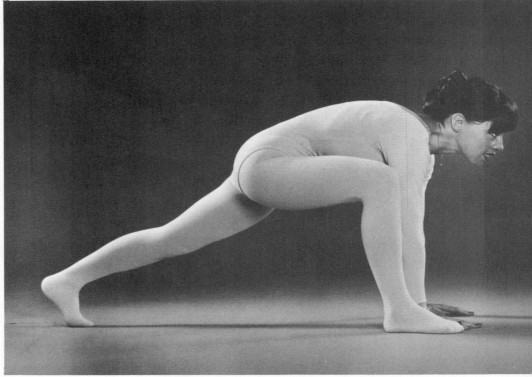

1

Beginning on your hands and feet, stretch your left leg out behind you so that it rests on the ball of the foot. Your right leg should be bent, with your right foot next to the outside of your right hand.

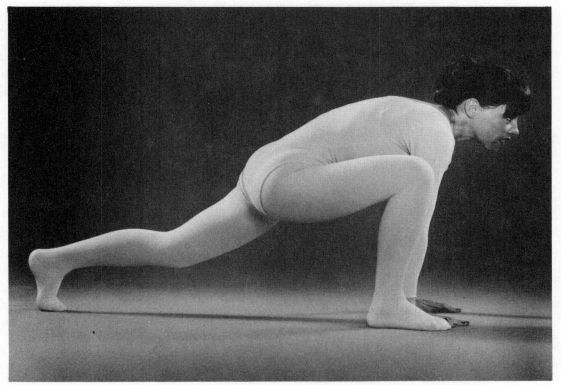

2

Rock your weight
forward, then back. Do
not allow your fanny to
stick up in the air, and
keep your right heel on
the floor.

SIDE SCISSORS

When you do this exercise, be sure your knees face forward and your legs are stretched to make them as long as possible.

To Reduce: complete sequence once

Maintenance: repeat sequence twice

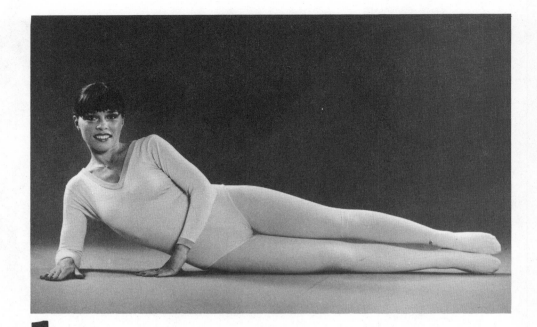

1

Lie on your right side with your torso propped up on your elbow. Keep your legs straight and your feet pointed. Your left arm should rest in front of you, with fingers on the floor for leverage.

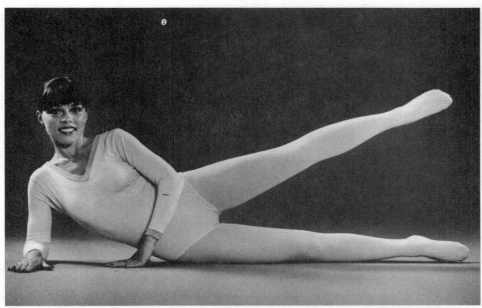

2

Raise and lower your left leg 8 times, keeping it stretched out and the foot pointed.

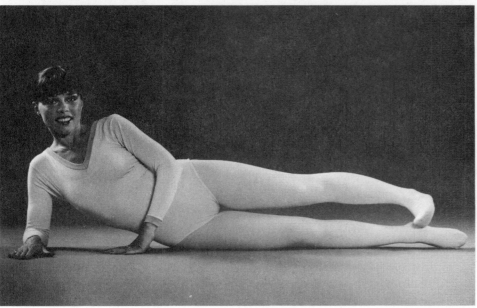

3

Flex your left foot, and raise and lower your left leg 8 more times, keeping it stretched out. Change sides and repeat the series with your right leg, first with foot pointed, then with foot flexed.

VERY DIFFICULT SIDE SCISSORS

When you keep your bottom leg raised 6 inches from the floor, this exercise will help tighten the inside of the bottom thigh and reduce the outside of the top thigh.

To Reduce: complete sequence once

Maintenance: repeat sequence twice

134

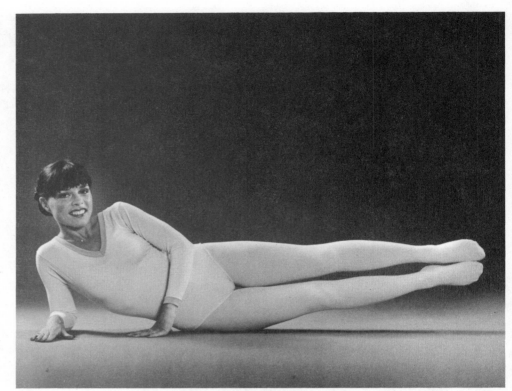

1

Lie on your right side with your torso propped up on your elbow and your left arm in front of you with fingers on the floor. Both legs should be straight, feet pointed, and raised about 6 inches from the floor. Stretch your legs and make them as long as possible.

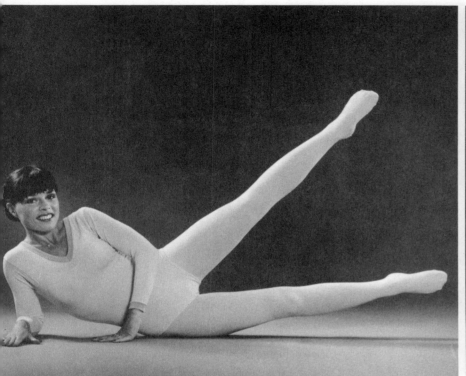 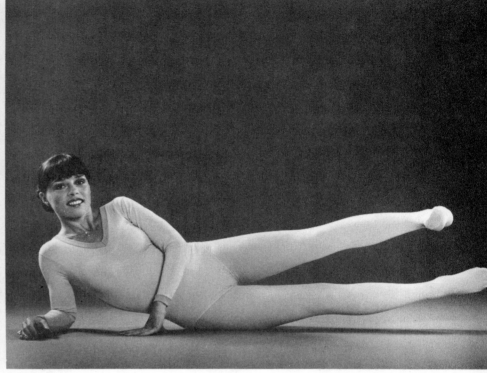

2

Raise and lower your left
leg 8 times, keeping it
stretched and your toes
pointed. Be sure your
right leg remains raised
from the floor.

3

Flex your left foot, and
raise and lower your left
leg 8 more times, still
keeping it stretched and
the bottom leg off the
floor. Change sides and
repeat the series with
your right leg.

135

ROCKETTE BEND AND KICK

This series of movements may seem confusing at first, but the combination of bending, lifting and lowering your leg acts to trim your thighs. You may want to turn your head to check the position of your knee and leg in the last steps of this exercise.

To Reduce: repeat 4 times with each leg

Maintenance: the same

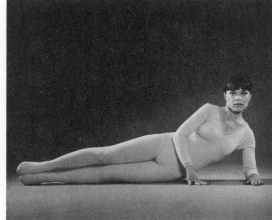

 1

Lie on your left side with your torso propped up on your left elbow and your right arm in front of you with fingers on the floor. Your legs should be straight and feet pointed.

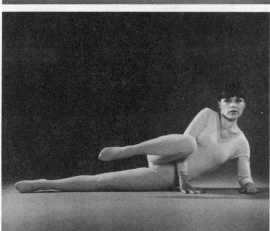

2

Bend your right leg, bringing the knee up to your chest. Your knee should face forward.

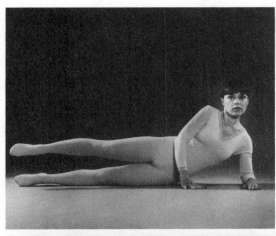

3

Straighten your leg, but do not allow it to rest on the left leg.

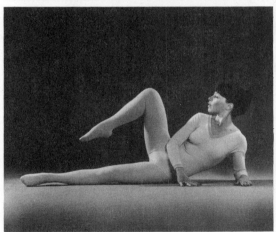

4

Bend your right leg again, this time bringing your knee up toward your shoulder. Your knee should face upward.

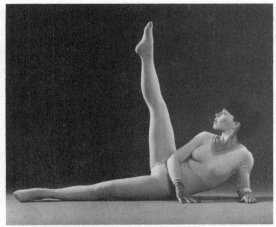

5

Straighten your right leg so it is perpendicular to your body.

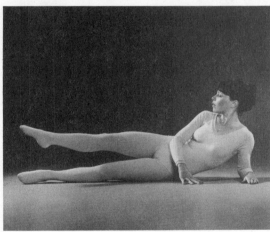

6

Slowly lower your right leg until it almost rests on your left leg. Your knee should still face the ceiling. Hold this position for 2 seconds. Turn the knee forward and lower the leg to the original position.

BATON LEG

Tightening your stomach and fanny muscles will help you keep your balance while your leg moves in a circle. Be sure to stretch out your legs during this exercise.

To Reduce: 4 times with each leg

Maintenance: 16 times with each leg, changing legs after 8

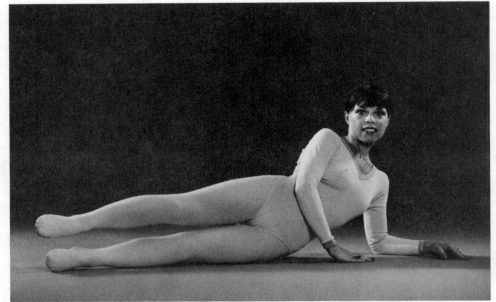

1

Lie on your left side with your torso propped up on your elbow. Your right arm should rest in front of you, with the palm of your hand on the floor. Your legs should be straight and your feet pointed. Raise your right leg 3 inches from the floor.

2

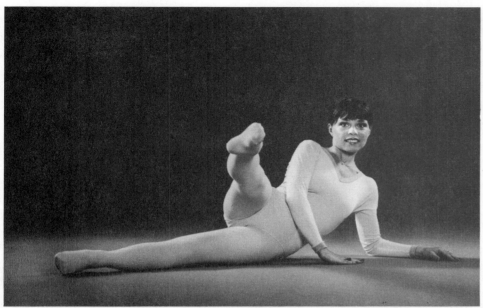

Swing your right leg forward, then back, keeping it straight and your torso still.

3

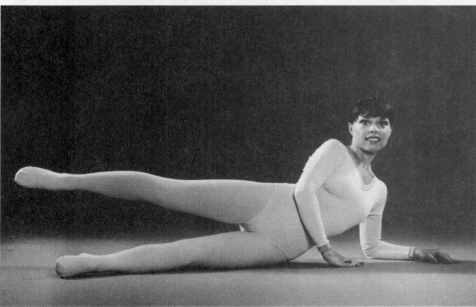

Without lowering your right leg, make 2 circles by moving it in a clockwise direction.

ORANGE JUICE SQUEEZE

When you first do this exercise, you may find it hard to lift your leg more than a few inches off the floor. After a few weeks, however, your legs will be stronger and the exercise easier.

To Reduce: complete sequence once on each side

Maintenance: the same

1

Lie on your left side with your torso propped up on your left elbow and your right arm resting in front. Your left palm should be flat on the floor. Bend your right leg so the ball of the right foot is on the floor behind your left knee. Keep your left leg straight.

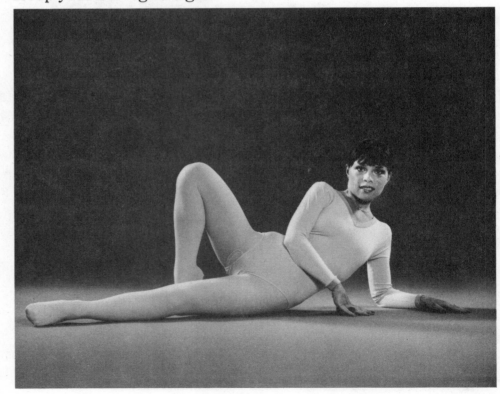

2

Keeping your right hip perpendicular to the floor, raise and lower your left leg 8 times, with the foot pointed. Lift the leg as high as you comfortably can, without leaning back on your fanny.

3

Flex your left foot, and raise and lower your left leg 8 times. Repeat the series with your right leg.

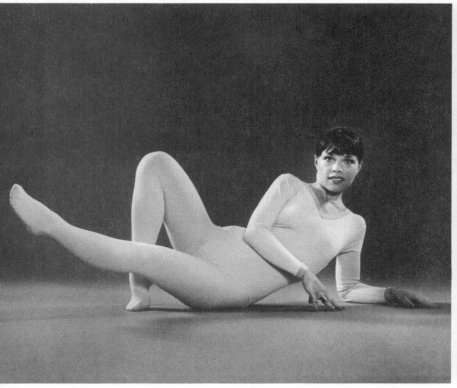

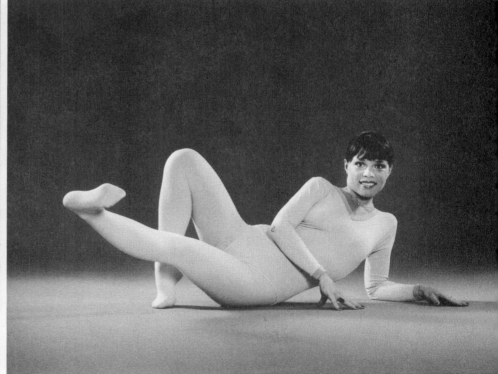

SPREAD EAGLE

Keep your lower back flat against the floor at all times so you don't strain it. When you raise and lower your leg, you'll feel the stretching of the muscles on the inside thigh.

To Reduce: complete sequence once with each leg

Maintenance: repeat sequence twice with each leg

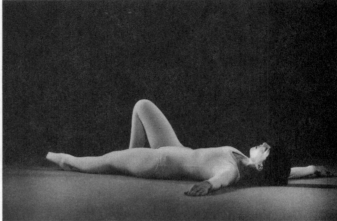

1

Lie flat on your back with arms stretched out. Your left leg should be straight, foot pointed, and your right leg bent with foot flat on the floor.

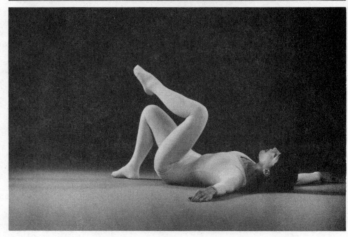

2

Raise your left leg, bending the knee in toward your chest.

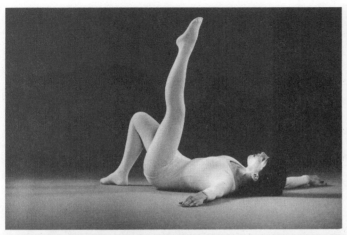

3

Straighten your leg so it is perpendicular to the floor. Keep your foot pointed.

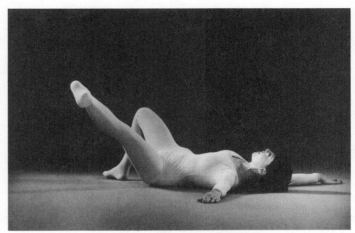

4

Slowly lower your left leg out to the side so it is parallel to your arm and within 10 inches of the floor. Raise and lower your left leg 8 times without resting it on the floor.

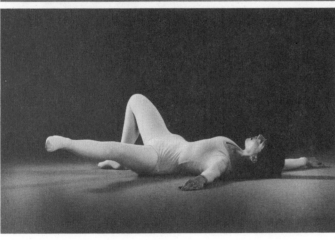

5

Flex your left foot, and raise and lower your left leg 8 more times. Repeat the series with your right leg.

ONE-SIDED TRIANGLE LIFT

The correct way to do this exercise is to make sure your body is completely vertical; this is harder than leaning over, but it will trim your thighs more effectively.

To Reduce: complete sequence once

Maintenance: repeat sequence twice

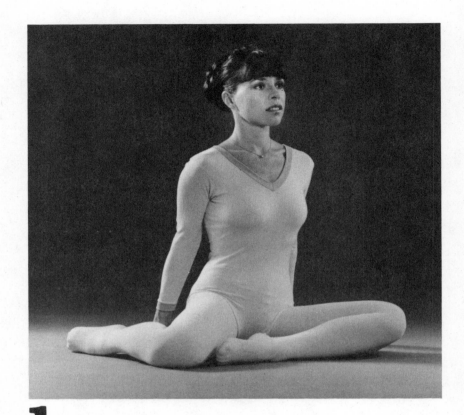

1

Sit with your left leg bent in front of you and your right leg bent to the side. Your left foot should touch your right knee, and your right foot should point backward. Place your hands on the floor behind your fanny.

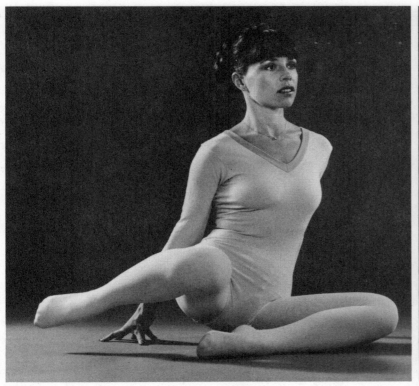

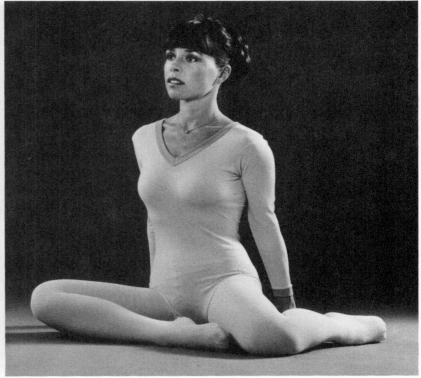

2

Raise and lower your
right leg 4 times, keeping
it bent. Keep your torso
as vertical as possible.

3

Reverse the position of
your legs and repeat the
exercise 4 times, lifting
your left leg.

STEM STIR

Make a large circle with your
leg for best results, and keep
your torso still.

To Reduce: complete
sequence once

Maintenance: repeat
sequence twice, resting your
leg between repetitions

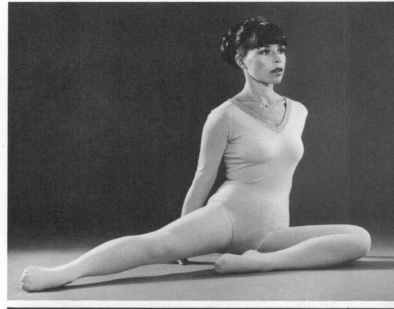

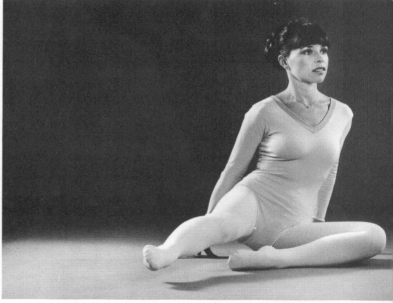

1

Sit with your left leg bent in front of you and your right leg stretched straight out to the side. Place your hands on the floor behind your fanny.

2

Raise your right leg several inches off the floor and bring it forward as far as you can.

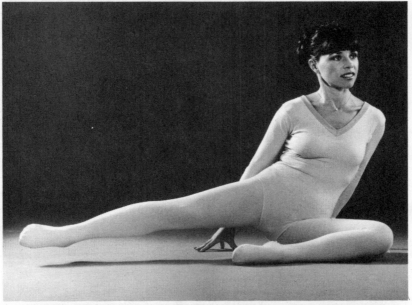

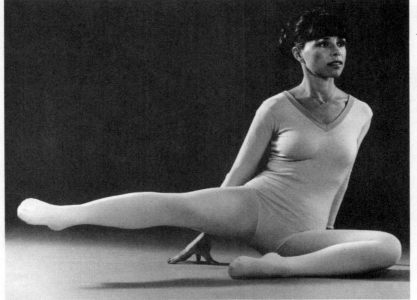

3

Lower your leg to within 2 inches of the floor, then swing it as far back as comfortably possible.

4

Complete the circle by bringing your right leg back to the original position; continue rotating your leg for a total of 4 times. Rotate 4 more times in the opposite direction, moving it backward, then down, then forward. Repeat the series with your left leg.

FIGURE 8 LEG SWING

You may have to bend your active leg when you first do this exercise, but try to keep it as straight as possible. After the first few weeks you should not have to bend it. Remember to keep your feet flexed. When you swing your active leg across the other, lead with your big toe; when you swing it back to the original position, lead with your little toe.

To Reduce: repeat sequence twice

Maintenance: the same

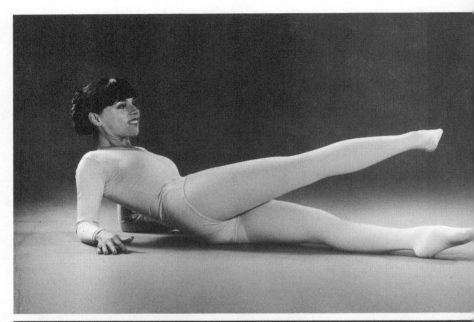

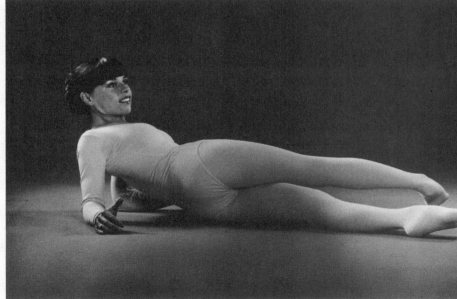

1

Lie on your back with your torso propped up on your arms and your legs stretched straight in front. Lift your right leg off the floor and flex your foot, turning it to the left.

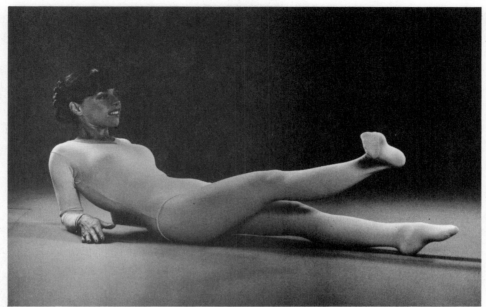

3

Turn the toes of your right foot to the right so it is still flexed but the toes point outward away from your body. Lift the leg and bring it back over your left leg to the front.

2

Swing your right leg over your left leg and touch the floor beyond it with your toes. Your fanny will leave the floor, but keep your upper body in its original position.

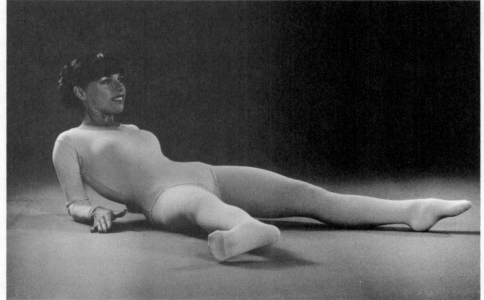

4

Lower your right leg so the little toe touches the floor and your legs are straight, spread apart in front of you. Swing your leg back and forth with flexed foot for a total of 8 times. Repeat the series with your left leg.

ON SHOULDERS, LEG SCISSORS

Move your legs slowly and smoothly, or you may lose your balance. When you finish the exercise, relax on the floor for 30 seconds to rest your shoulders.

To Reduce: complete sequence once, opening and crossing your legs 16 times

Maintenance: complete sequence once, opening and crossing your legs 24 times, if comfortable

150

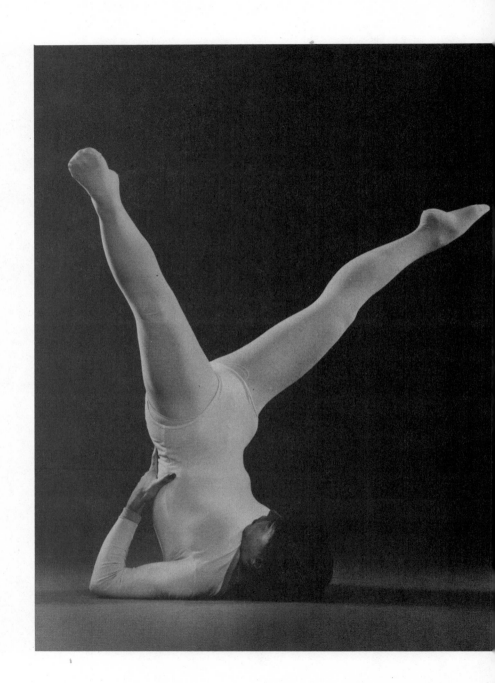

1

Lie flat on your back, bend your knees, and bring your legs up over your head. Lift them straight in the air so your fanny and back are off the floor and your weight rests on your shoulders. Support your back with your hands (see Toe Dipping). Spread your legs as far apart as you can, keeping them straight and pointing your feet. Your knees should face outward.

2

Bring your legs together and cross them without bending your knees. Open and cross your legs 16 times.

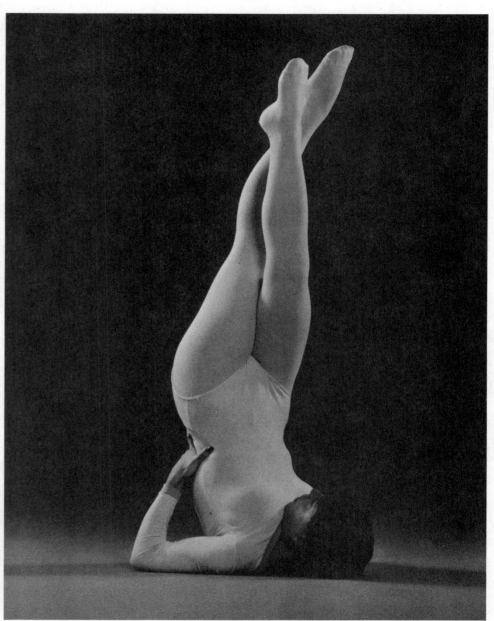

FIRE HYDRANT

When your leg is raised and stretched to the side, your hip will also be raised. But when you lift your leg behind you, both hips should be parallel to the floor.

To Reduce: repeat sequence 6 times with each leg

Maintenance: repeat sequence 12 times with each leg, changing legs after 6

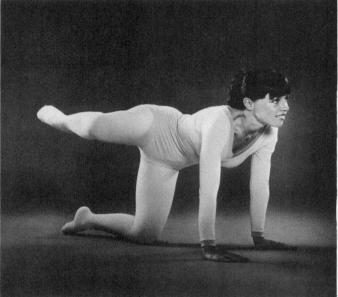

1

Starting on your hands and knees, raise your right leg in a bent position so your thigh is parallel to the floor and your foot points straight behind you.

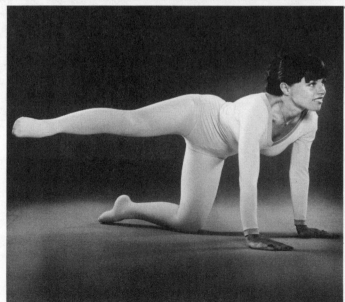

2

Straighten your leg, keeping the thigh in the same position. Your right leg will be parallel to the floor, with the knee facing forward.

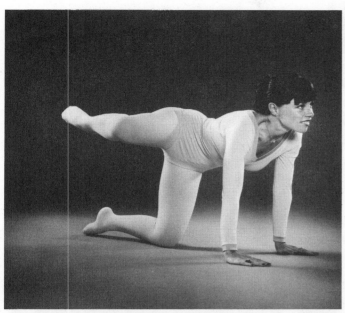

3

Bend your knee to bring the leg to the original position.

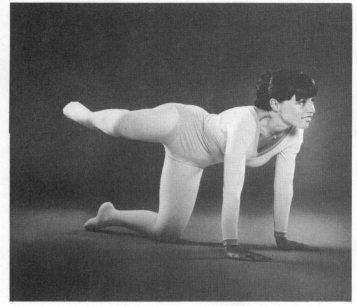

4

Straighten your leg, kicking it out behind you. Your knee will face the floor.

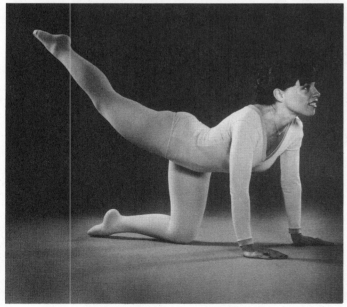

5

Bring your leg back to the original bent position, and straighten it out to the side. Return your leg to the bent position once more before lowering it to the floor.

CALVES & ANKLES

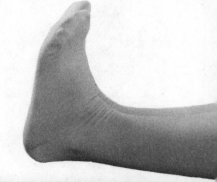

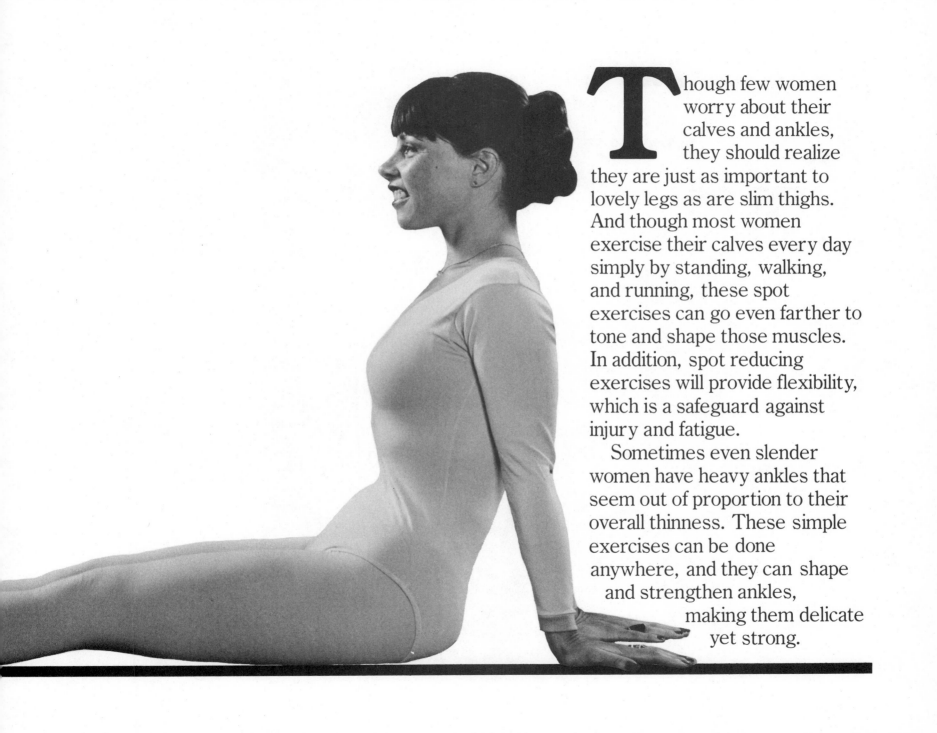

Though few women worry about their calves and ankles, they should realize they are just as important to lovely legs as are slim thighs. And though most women exercise their calves every day simply by standing, walking, and running, these spot exercises can go even farther to tone and shape those muscles. In addition, spot reducing exercises will provide flexibility, which is a safeguard against injury and fatigue.

Sometimes even slender women have heavy ankles that seem out of proportion to their overall thinness. These simple exercises can be done anywhere, and they can shape and strengthen ankles, making them delicate yet strong.

CALVES AND ANKLES

THE MIME'S WALK

Raise and lower your heels as slowly as you can for best results.

To Reduce: repeat sequence 16 times

Maintenance: repeat sequence 32 times

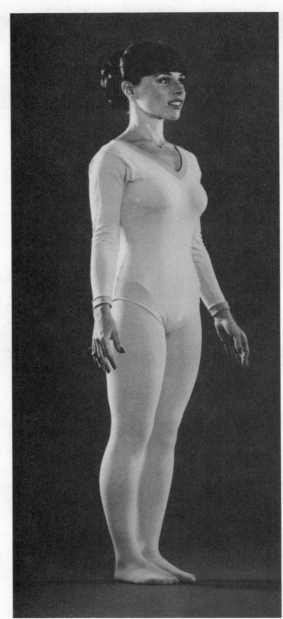

1

Stand with your legs straight, feet together, and arms relaxed at your sides. Tighten your stomach and fanny muscles.

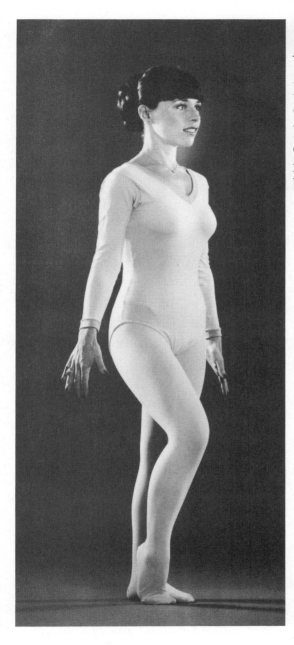

2

Raise your right heel, leaving only the ball of your right foot on the floor. Your right knee will bend slightly.

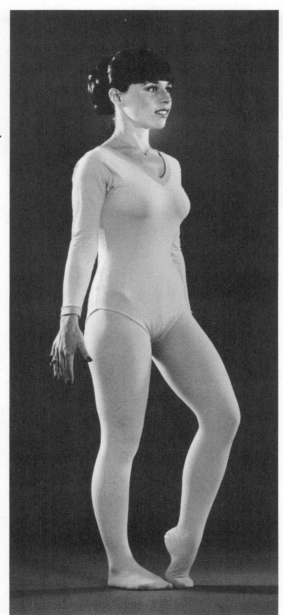

3

With a slow, steady motion, lower your right heel and lift your left heel off the floor. Raise and lower your heels in alternation.

GROWING

You must not hold on to a chair for balance during this exercise; if you do, it will be much less effective.

To Reduce: repeat sequence 4 times, counting slowly to 8

Maintenance: repeat sequence 6 times, counting to 10

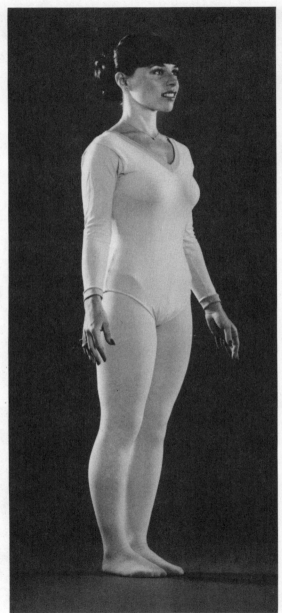

1

Stand with your legs straight, feet together, and arms relaxed at your sides. Tighten your stomach and fanny muscles.

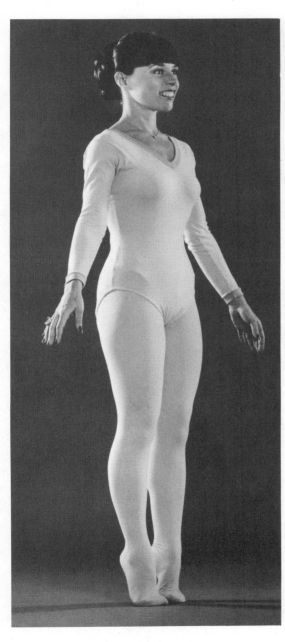

2

Rise slowly onto
the balls of your
feet and maintain
this position for 2
seconds.

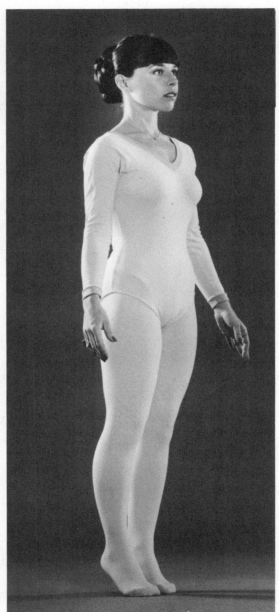

3

Slowly lower
your heels to the
floor.

159

CALVES AND ANKLES

TIPTOE BEND

Keep your back straight and your fanny muscles tightened as you do this exercise; you may hold on to a chair if you feel it's necessary.

To Reduce: 12 knee bends

Maintenance: 18 knee bends

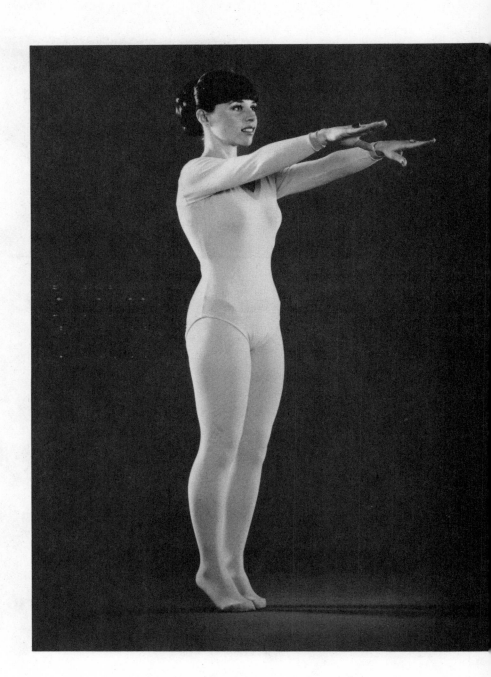

1

Stand with your legs straight, feet together, and arms stretched out in front at shoulder height. Rise onto the balls of your feet.

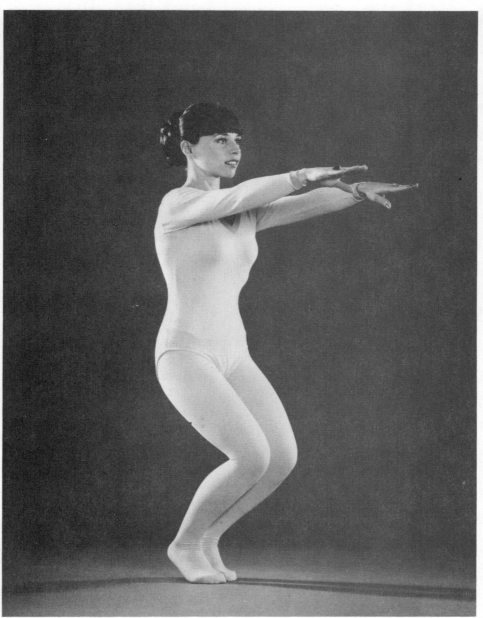

2

Bend your knees, lowering your torso about 12 inches. Do not lower your heels. Straighten your legs, but stay on the balls of your feet. Be sure to keep your stomach and fanny muscles tightened.

ROPE JUMPING

Rope jumping is excellent for trimming calves. Any rope—it doesn't have to be a "professional" jump rope—will do, but its two ends should touch your armpits when you stand in the middle of it.

To Reduce: 10 seconds of jumping

Maintenance: work up to 3 or 4 minutes

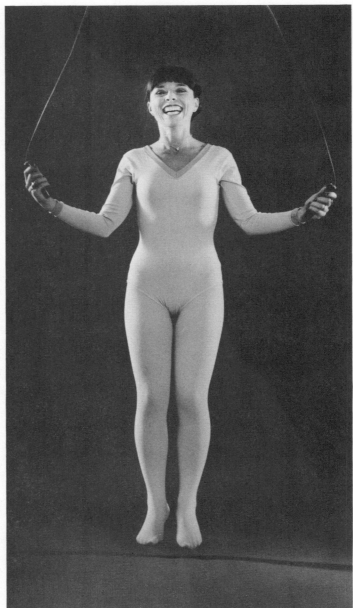

1

Jump rope with your feet together and knees bent slightly, starting with 10 seconds of jumping. Work up to 3 or 4 minutes in 4 weeks.

FLEXIBLE FEET

Don't be fooled by the simplicity of this exercise; it does stretch and trim the calf muscles. The exercise can also be done with your legs slightly raised off the floor.

To Reduce: repeat sequence 16 times

Maintenance: repeat sequence 24 times

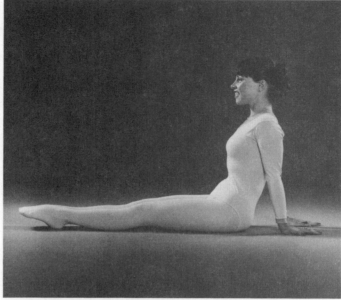

1

Sit on the floor with your legs stretched straight in front and your hands on the floor behind your fanny. Point your feet as far forward as you can.

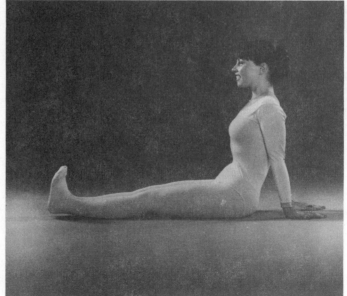

2

Flex your feet, pointing them back up toward your body and lifting your heels off the floor.

163

ANKLE CIRCLE

Some people swing their feet around in a circle when they're impatient; by doing this slowly you can trim your ankles.

To Reduce: complete sequence once

Maintenance: repeat sequence twice

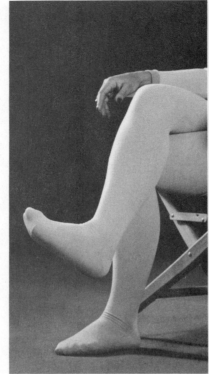

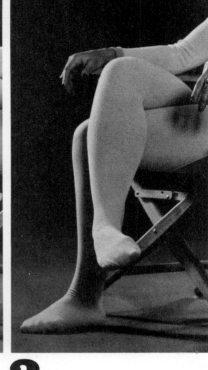

1

Sit in a chair and cross your right leg over your left. Flex your right foot and rotate it from the ankle in 4 clockwise circles.

2

Move your foot in 4 counter-clockwise circles. Reverse the position of your legs and circle your flexed left foot 4 times in each direction.

POINT AND FLEX

For best results, point and flex your foot as far as you can; see if you can make a straight line of your foot and shin when your foot is pointed.

To Reduce: complete sequence once

Maintenance: complete sequence once, pointing and flexing your foot 24 times

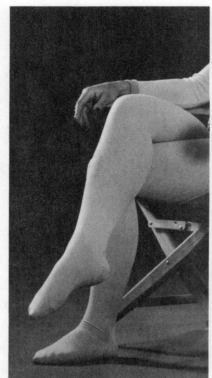

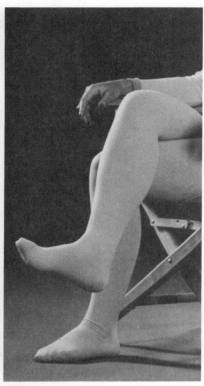

1

Sit in a chair and cross your right leg over your left. Point your foot downward as far as possible.

2

Flex your right foot, pointing it back up toward your body. Point and flex the foot 16 times, then reverse the position of your legs. Point and flex your left foot 16 times.

TWIST AGAIN

This is a particularly good exercise to do to lively music. Be sure to keep your stomach and fanny muscles tightened and your back straight.

To Reduce: repeat sequence 8 times

Maintenance: repeat sequence 12 times

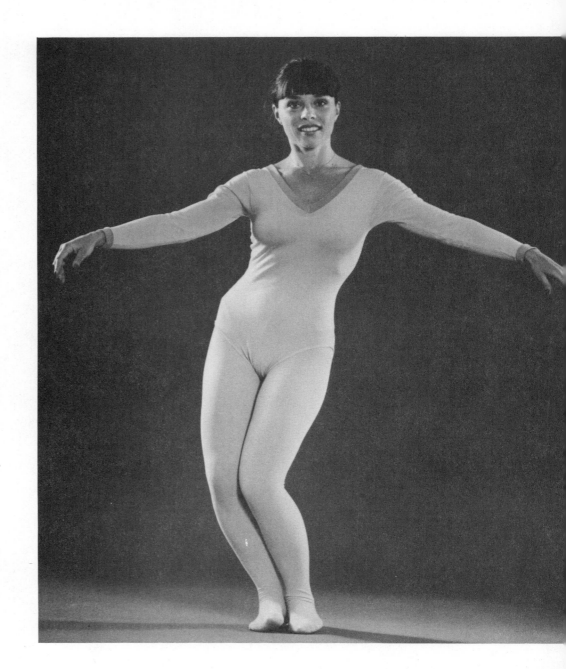

1

Stand with your legs straight, feet together, and arms raised from your sides. Bend your knees slightly and twist them to the right so your weight is on the outside of your right foot and the inside of your left foot.

2

Turn your knees to the left so your weight rests on the outside of your left foot and the inside of your right foot. Twist back and forth, keeping your back straight.

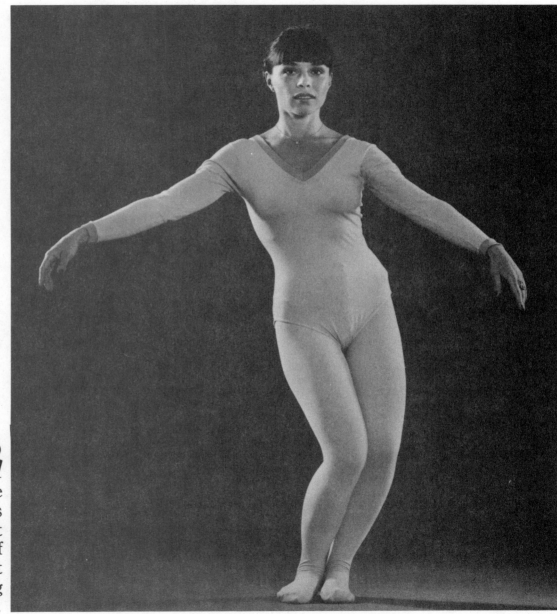

CURLED TOES

When your feet are curled, there should be a hollow half-circle between them and the floor.

To Reduce: repeat sequence 6 times

Maintenance: repeat sequence 9 times

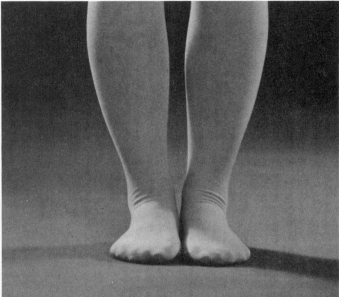

1

Stand with your legs straight, feet together, and arms at your sides. Tighten your stomach and fanny muscles.

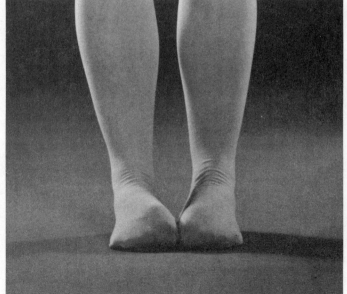

2

Curl your toes under and your insteps out so your weight rests on the outsides of your feet. Flatten your feet, bringing them back to the original position.

LOWERING HEELS

You may want to hold the back of a chair for balance. Be careful not to lower your heels so far that you strain them; stop if you feel any pain.

To Reduce: repeat sequence 8 times

Maintenance: repeat sequence 16 times

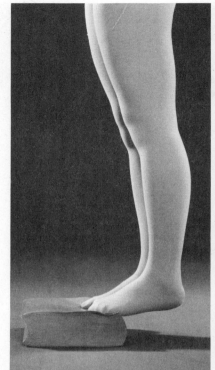

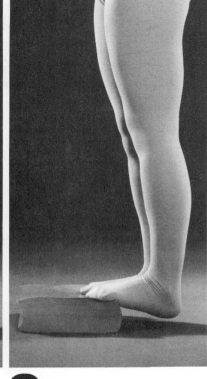

1

Stand straight on a thick book such as a dictionary or phone book. Only the balls of your feet (not your heels) should be supported by the book.

2

Lower your heels as far toward the floor as you comfortably can. Hold the lowered position for 8 seconds, then lift your heels to the original position.

FLEXIBILITY

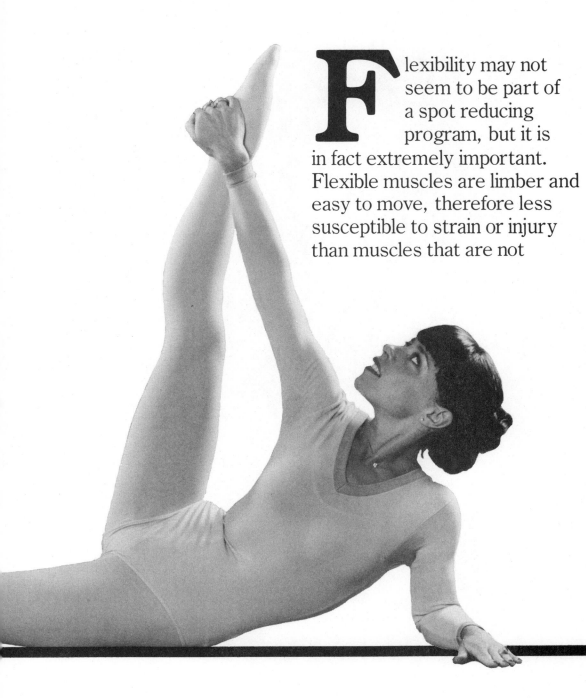

Flexibility may not seem to be part of a spot reducing program, but it is in fact extremely important. Flexible muscles are limber and easy to move, therefore less susceptible to strain or injury than muscles that are not flexible. Though the spot reducing exercises in this book strengthen and tone various sets of muscles, you will achieve overall flexibility through different series of movements. Most important, your muscles will become long and lean, rather than short and bulky, giving your body the graceful slimness you want.

You should end each exercise session with several of these routines, to relax and gently stretch the muscles you've been exerting. As your flexibility increases, you'll be able to move more freely and gracefully—not only during exercise sessions, but throughout the day.

RAG DOLL

When you finish this exercise, bring your head up slowly so that you don't get dizzy. Don't stretch too far or you may strain your back.

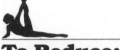

To Reduce: repeat sequence 3 times

Maintenance: the same

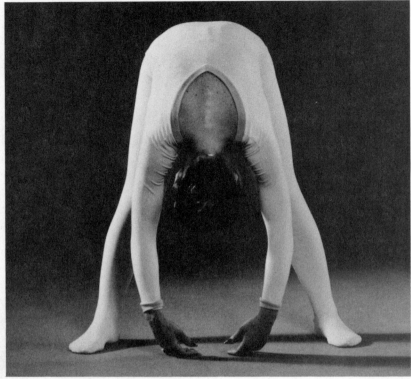

1

Stand with your legs straight, feet apart, and torso bent forward from the hips. Let your arms dangle in front of you. Bounce your torso toward the floor 8 times.

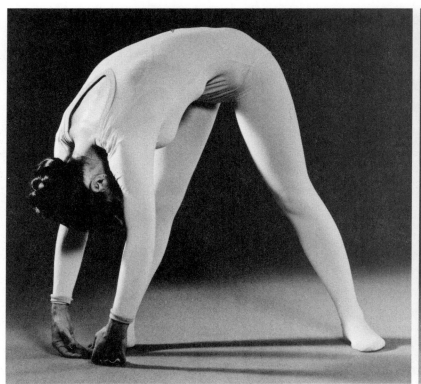

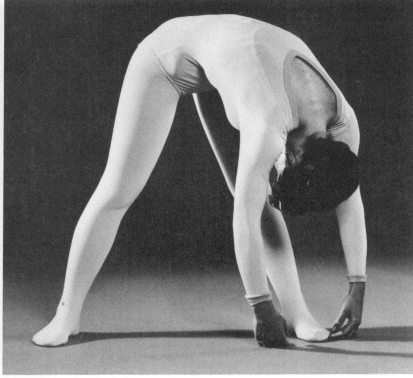

2

Turn your torso over
your right leg and bounce
8 times. Keep both legs
straight.

3

Turn your torso over
your left leg and bounce 8
times.

TWIST AND PECK

Although this exercise looks complicated, the movements are actually simple. Keep your arms straight and raised as high as possible above your back.

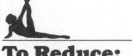

To Reduce: repeat sequence 8 times

Maintenance: repeat sequence 16 times

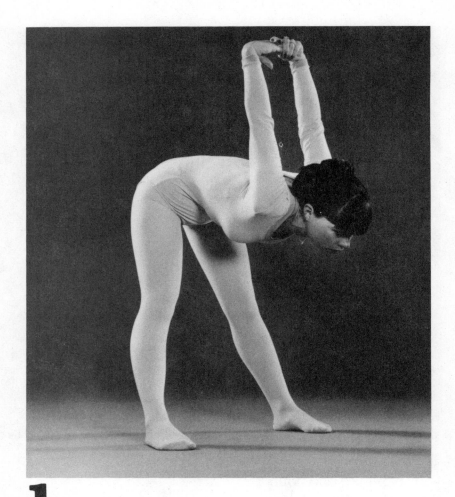

1

Stand with your feet apart and your torso bent forward from the hips. Keeping your knees straight, clasp your hands behind your back and raise them as high as you can.

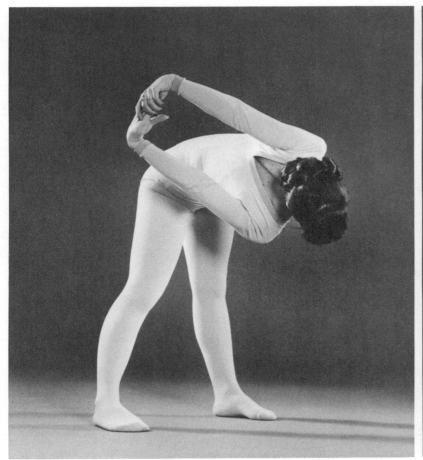 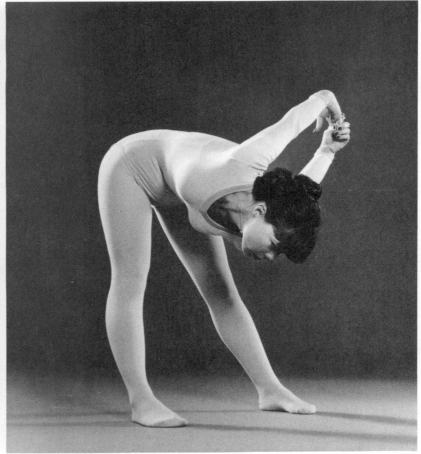

2

Twist your right shoulder down, and lift your left shoulder up and back. In this position, lower your torso toward the floor, leading with your right shoulder.

3

Twist your left shoulder, lifting your right shoulder up and back. Lower your torso toward the floor again, this time leading with your left shoulder.

CLOSING DOWN

This is not a bouncing exercise; you must stretch slowly and carefully. When you finish, shake and bend your legs to relax them.

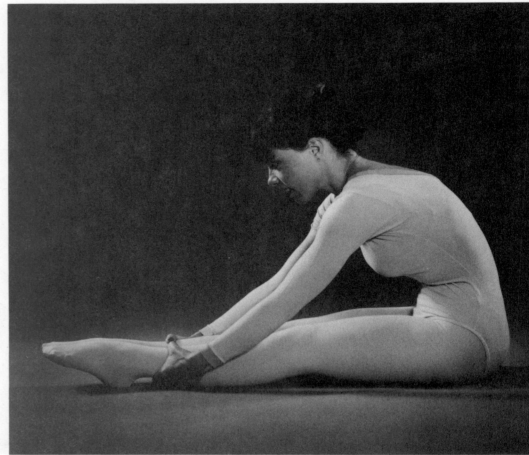

To Reduce: repeat 6 times

Maintenance: repeat 12 times

1

Sit on the floor with your legs together, stretched straight out in front of you. Hold your calves with your hands.

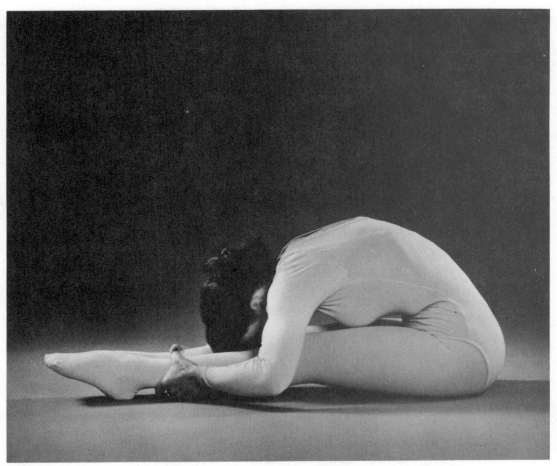

2

Slowly pull your torso
forward, bringing it as
close to your thighs as
you can. Hold this
position for 8 seconds,
then release.

SITTING "C"

The effectiveness of this exercise depends on not bending forward at the waist. Your upper shoulder should be thrust slightly backward in order to keep your torso straight.

To Reduce: repeat sequence 3 times

Maintenance: the same

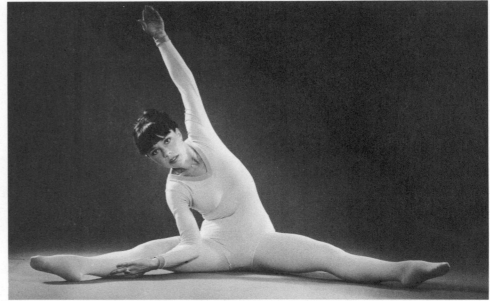

1

Sit on the floor with your legs straight and spread as far apart as possible in front of you, with your knees facing the ceiling and feet pointed. Keep your torso upright and face forward. Place the palm of your right hand facing upward beneath your right calf, and raise your left arm straight over your head.

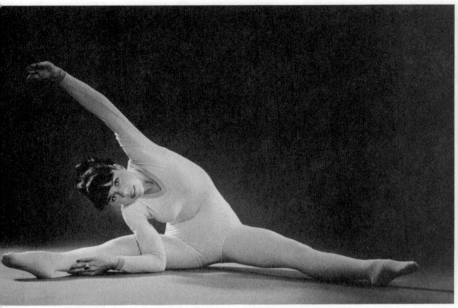

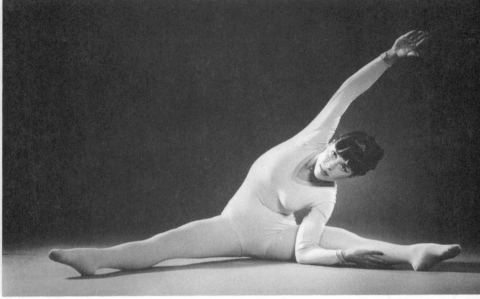

2

Stretch your left arm to
the right, making an arc
of your body. Bounce
your torso and arm 8
times to the right. Do not
lower your left shoulder
and be sure to continue
to face forward.

3

Reverse the position of
your arms so your left
palm is facing upward
under your left calf and
your right arm is raised
over your head. Stretch
your arm and torso to the
left without lowering
your right shoulder, and
bounce 8 times.

MEDITATION

Do this exercise slowly; it is meant to relax and stretch your body comfortably. Only lower your torso as far as you can, and do not force your elbows down. After a few weeks your flexibility will improve.

To Reduce: repeat 4 times

Maintenance: repeat 8 times

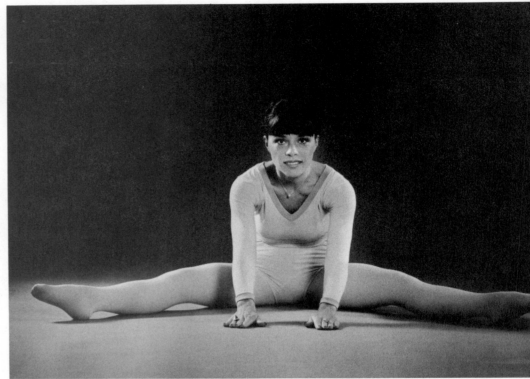

1

Sit on the floor with your legs straight and spread as far apart as possible. Your feet should be pointed and your knees facing the ceiling. Bend your torso forward and place the palms of your hands flat on the floor about 18 inches in front of you.

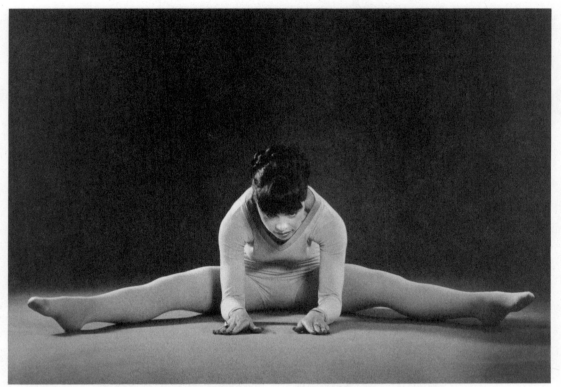

2

Slowly lower your torso
as far forward as you can
and lower your elbows to
the floor. Hold this
position for 12 seconds,
then relax.

UNFOLDING

The movements in this sequence should be performed as smoothly as possible once the exercise becomes familiar. It's very good for all-over suppleness.

To Reduce: repeat sequence 6 times

Maintenance: repeat sequence 10–12 times

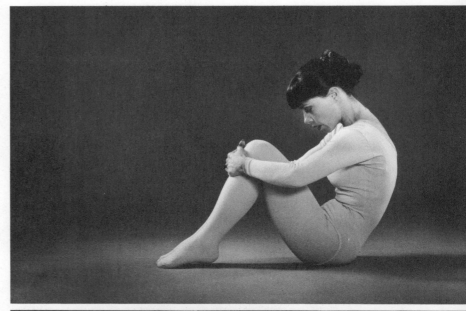

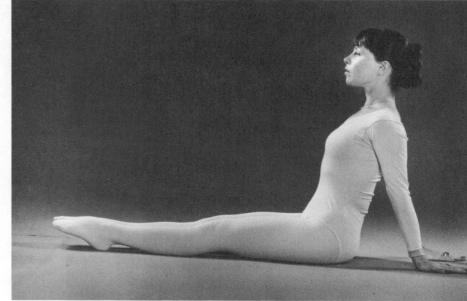

1

Sit on the floor with your knees bent and together, and your hands clasped around them. Keep your feet flat on the floor. Pull in your stomach, round your back, and tilt your head forward.

2

Place your hands on the floor behind your fanny and stretch your legs out straight in front of you, feet together and pointed. Arch your back slightly.

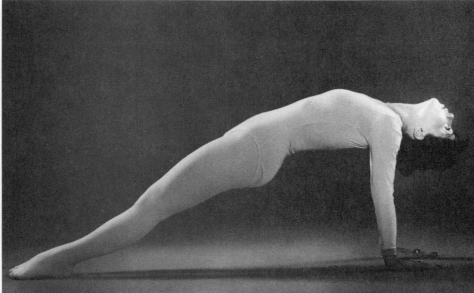

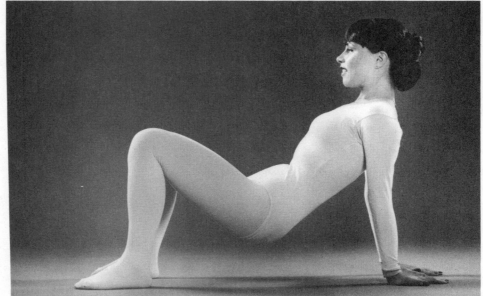

3

Lift your fanny off the floor and straighten your torso. Your body should form a slight arch from feet to chin. Stretch your neck and allow your head to fall back. Hold this position for 4 seconds.

4

Lower your torso and fanny to the original sitting position.

THE "L" SHAPED BODY

It may be too difficult at first to straighten your leg all the way while holding the foot in your hand. If so, hold your calf and try to stretch a little farther each time you do the exercise. In a few weeks you'll be able to hold your foot.

To Reduce: repeat sequence 5 times with each leg from step 2

Maintenance: the same, but pull your leg as close as possible to your body

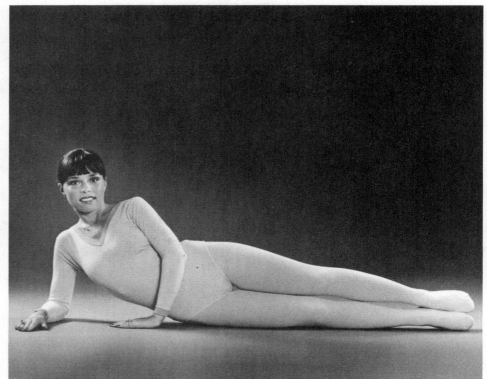

1

Lie on your right side with your torso propped up on your elbow and your left hand resting in front. Your legs should be straight with feet pointed.

184

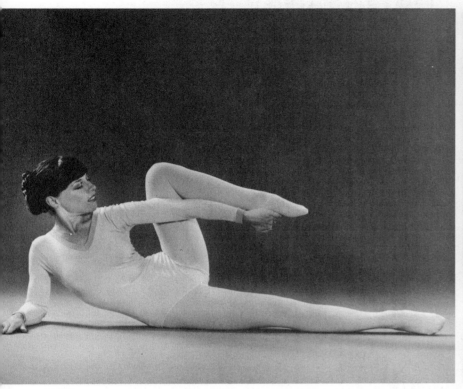

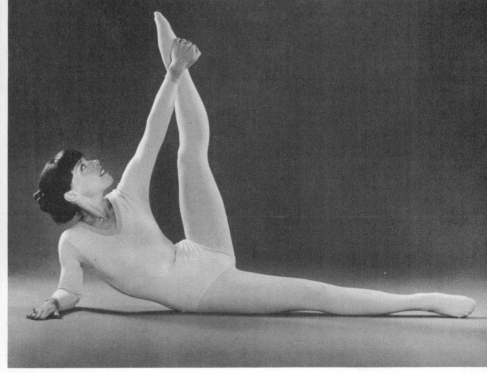

2

Bend your left leg, and
with your left hand clasp
the arch of the foot. Your
elbow should be next to
the inner thigh, and your
knee facing the ceiling.

3

Still holding your right
foot, straighten the leg so
it is perpendicular to the
floor. Hold this position
for 4 seconds, then bend
the knee.

BOTTOMS UP

Be careful not to strain as you do this exercise; lift your fanny slowly and only as far as you comfortably can. You should feel a pulling sensation in the backs of your legs, but stop if you feel pain.

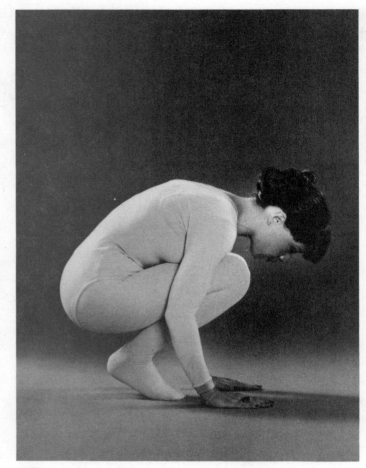

To Reduce: repeat 8 times

Maintenance: repeat 12 times

1

Crouch with your weight on your hands and toes so your knees are between your arms. Your palms should be flat on the floor in front of your feet.

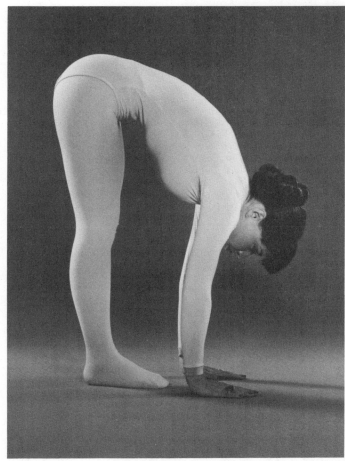

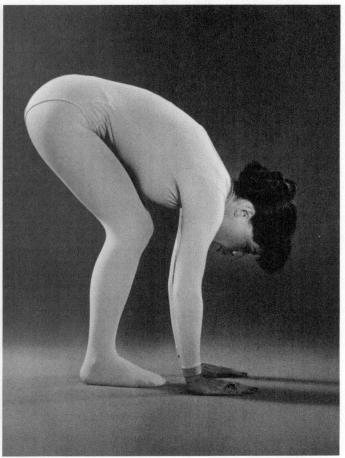

2

Slowly straighten your legs, lifting your fanny in the air.

3

Keep your fanny raised for 5 seconds, then return to the original position.

RUBBER WOMAN

Your goal should be to lower your head all the way to your knees, but it will probably take you a while to reach that degree of flexibility. Don't force yourself; you risk injuring your back.

To Reduce: repeat 4 to 6 times

Maintenance: repeat 8 times

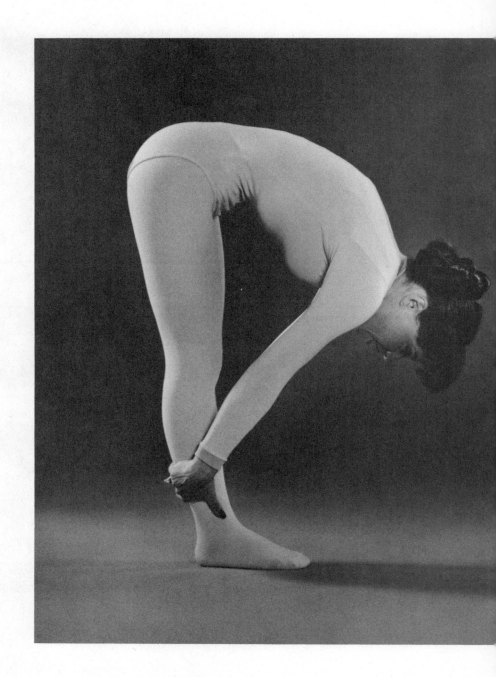

1

Stand with your feet together and your legs straight. Bend forward so that both hands can easily clasp your calves.

2

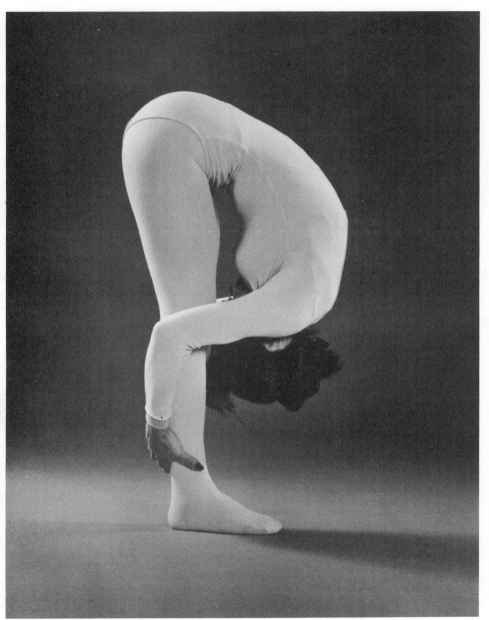

Keeping your knees straight, slowly pull your head and torso in as far as you can toward your legs. Hold this position for 8 seconds, then release it.

THE CHOREO-GRAPHED STRETCH

This exercise may seem long and complicated at first, but as you learn the order of the movements you'll be able to perform them smoothly. You should always end your exercise session with this stretch, which will loosen your muscles and leave your entire body thoroughly relaxed.

To Reduce: repeat sequence 6 times

Maintenance: the same

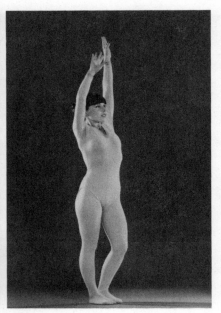

1

Stand with your legs straight, feet together, and arms stretched straight up above your head.

2

Bend your left knee slightly and stretch your left arm over your head. Straighten your left knee and relax your left arm, but don't lower it. Repeat with the right side. Stretch each arm 8 times, alternating.

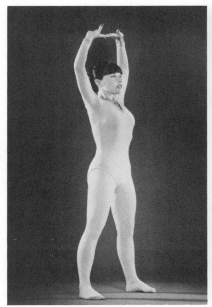
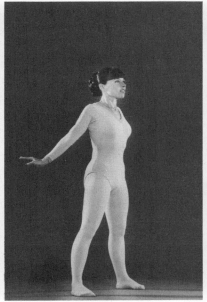
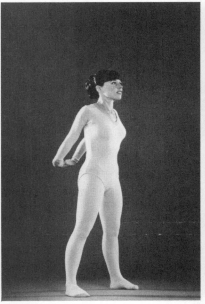
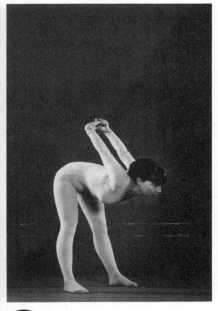

3

Spread your feet
apart and arch
your arms over
your head so the
tips of your
fingers touch
and your palms
face upward. Do
not arch your
back.

4

Pull your hands
apart, and lower
your arms to a
count of 4. Keep
your hands
pointing upward.

5

Clasp your hands
tightly behind
your fanny.

6

Bend your torso
forward from the
hips, raising your
arms as high as
you can above
your back.
Bounce forward
4 times.

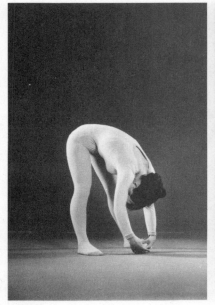 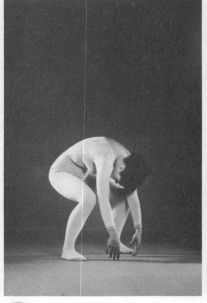 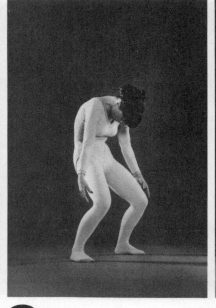 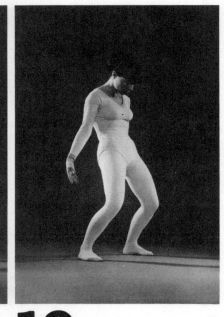

7

Unclasp your hands and let your arms dangle in front of your legs. Bounce forward with straight legs 4 times.

8

Bend your knees and tuck your pelvis forward.

9

Slowly straighten your torso, keeping your knees bent.

10

As your body straightens, your hands should fall behind your fanny.

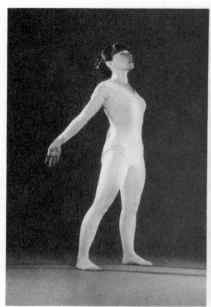

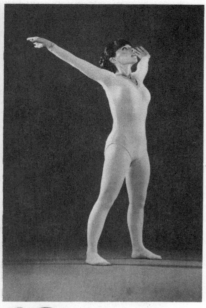

11

Straighten your
legs, stretch
your arms
behind you, and
arch your upper
back.

12

Raise your
straight arms
over your head
and bring your
feet together.
This will bring
you to the
original starting
position.

MAN'S
STYLE

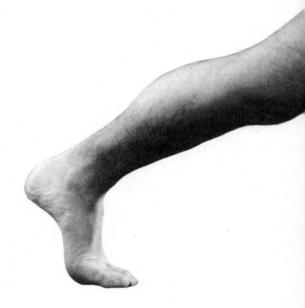

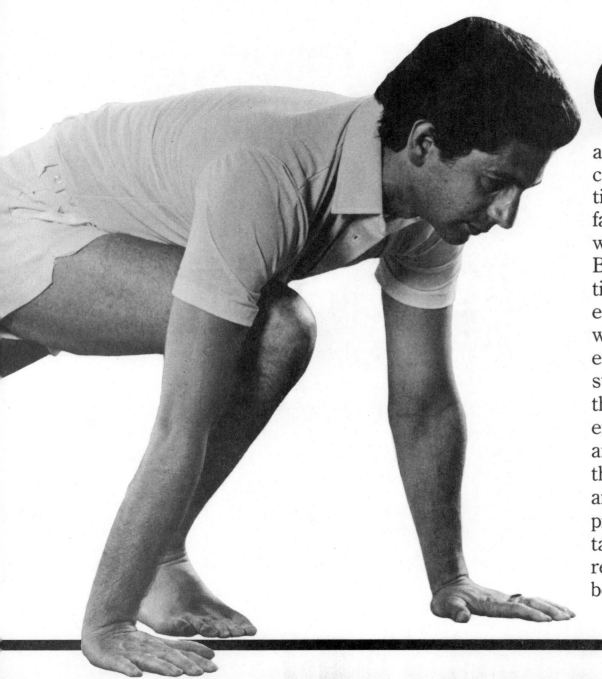

One of the first signs of age in men is the development of excess flab around the midsection, often called "love handles" or "a spare tire." Men seem to accumulate fat around their waist the way women do around their thighs. But simple dieting and a little time devoted to spot reducing exercises can make that extra weight disappear. The following exercises will stretch and strengthen the muscles around the waist and midriff to firm the entire midsection. Also included are several exercises for legs that will stretch the hamstrings and strengthen the thighs. This program for men, without taking much time, can quickly result in a fit and handsome body.

CLASSIC SIT-UP

This familiar exercise is one of the best for quickly trimming a flabby stomach. Be sure your stomach muscles are pulled in throughout.

To Reduce: complete 4 sit-ups

Maintenance: add 4 sit-ups per week, working up to 24

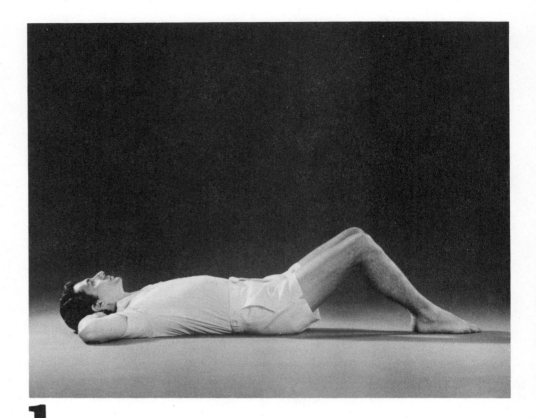

1

Lie flat on your back with knees bent and feet flat on the floor. Clasp your hands behind your neck.

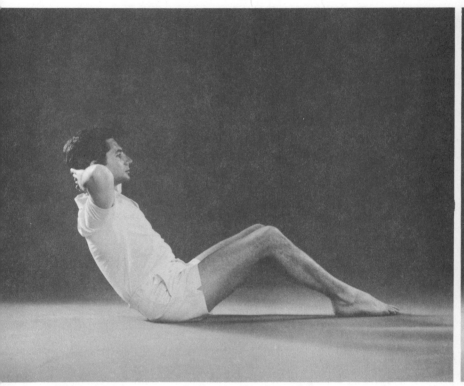

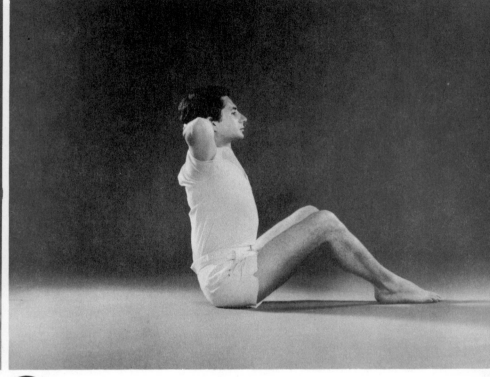

2

Slowly bring your torso
up into a sitting position,
with your back rounded.
Keep your feet flat on the
floor.

3

When you reach a sitting
position, straighten your
back, keeping your
stomach pulled in. Hold.
Round your back and
lower your torso slowly
to the floor.

PELICAN TWIST

To prevent dizziness, look at the floor while you twist your torso. Do not exceed 16 twists, or you may strain your muscles.

To Reduce: repeat sequence 8 times

Maintenance: the same

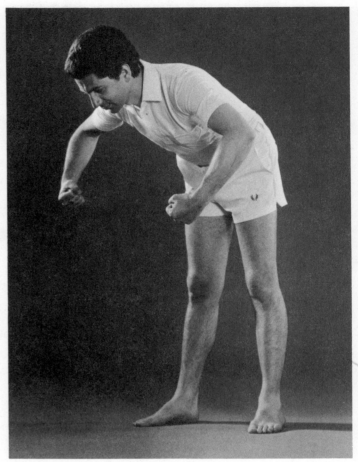

1

Stand straight with your feet apart. Bend forward at the hips but keep your back straight. Make your hands into fists and bend your arms. Your fists should almost meet in front of your chest.

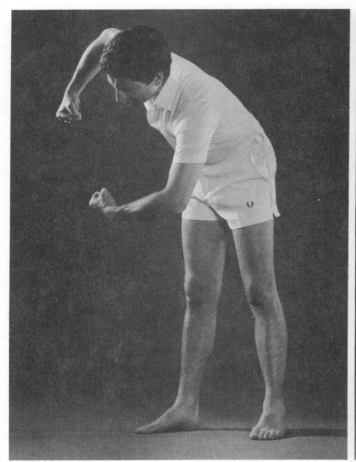

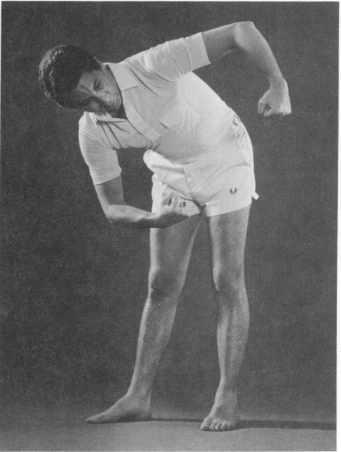

2

Twist your torso up to the
right, keeping your arms in
their original position. Your
right elbow should point
toward the ceiling, your left
elbow toward the floor.

3

Reverse the position of
your body, twisting your
torso up to the left and
raising your left elbow.
Twist back and forth,
always looking at the floor.

199

COPTER TWIST

It's important to allow only your upper body to move while you do this exercise, and to twist your body as far as you can in each direction.

To Reduce: repeat sequence 8 times

Maintenance: repeat sequence 16 times

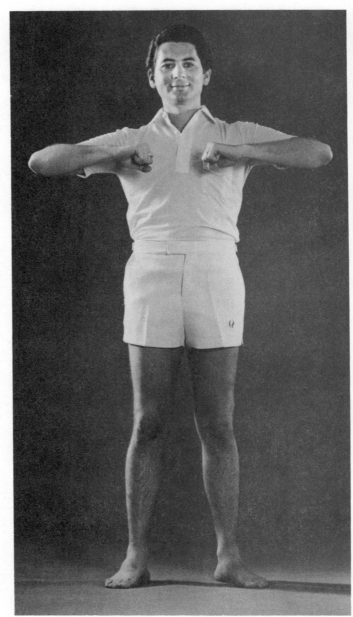

1

Stand straight with feet apart and arms bent at chest level, with your upper arms raised slightly away from the body. Make your hands into fists.

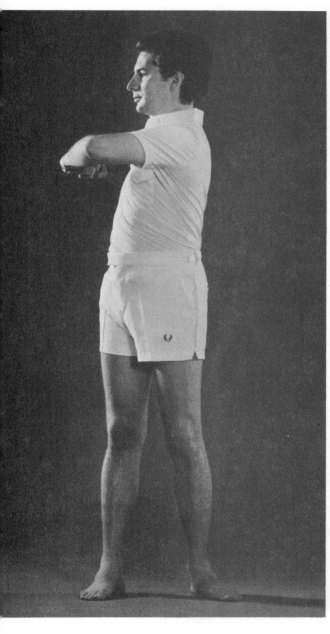

2

Without moving
your hips or
lower body, twist
your torso twice
to the right as
far as you can.

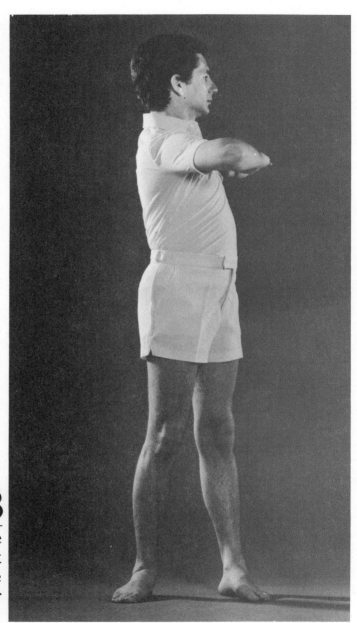

3

In the same
manner, twist
your torso twice
to the left as far
as you can.

ELASTIC "C"

When you do this exercise correctly, you'll feel the muscles stretch along your waist and ribs. Do not lean forward or arch your back; be careful to bend directly sideways.

To Reduce: complete sequence twice

Maintenance: repeat sequence 3 times

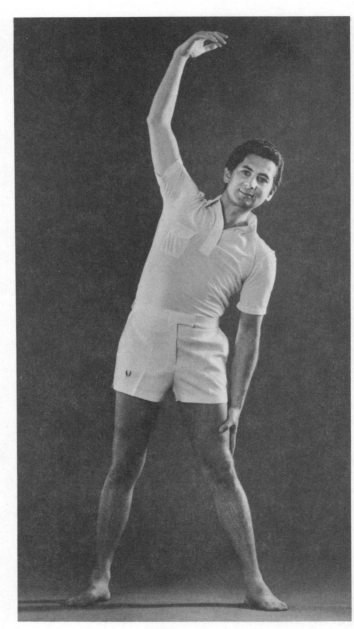

1

Stand straight with your feet apart, and stretch your right arm over your head, leaving your left arm relaxed at your side. Curve your torso to the left without bending forward or arching your back. Reach as far to the left as you can with your right arm.

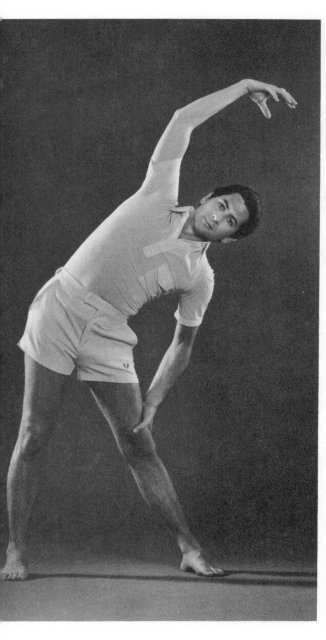

2

Bounce to the
left 8 times,
stretching your
right arm as far
as possible
without bending
your back or
twisting your
torso. Keep your
left arm relaxed
at your side.

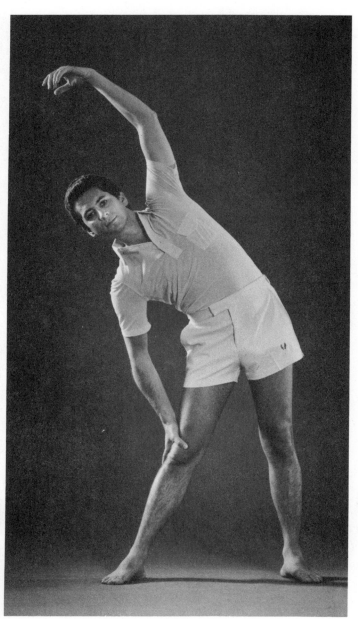

3

Reverse arms
and bounce 8
times to the
right.

DOWEL TWIST

You may not be able to keep your arms perfectly straight as you lower the dowel behind your back until after a few weeks of doing this exercise. Bend your arms only when you cannot lower them farther in the straight position. Keep your back straight, not arched, and your stomach muscles tightened. (You may use a broomstick in place of a dowel.)

To Reduce: complete sequence once

Maintenance: the same

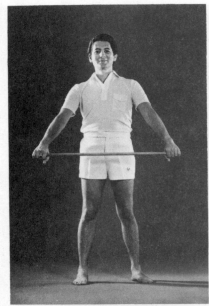

1

Stand with your feet apart and your legs straight, holding a dowel (¾ inch in diameter) in front of you with hands 3 feet apart, just below your hips.

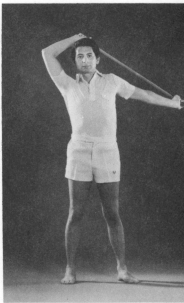

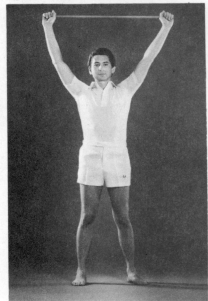

2

Without bending your arms, raise the dowel up over your head.

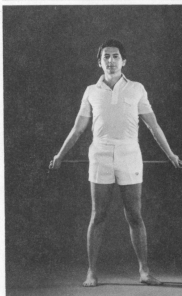

3

Lower the dowel behind you, keeping your arms straight as far as possible. You may have to bend your arms when you first do this exercise, but be sure to maintain the position of your hands.

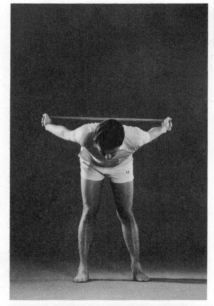

4

Lower the dowel to about 6 inches behind your fanny. Your arms should be straight.

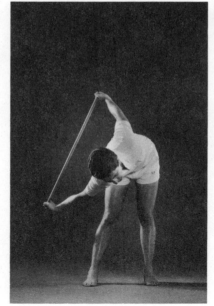

5

Bend forward at the hips without rounding your back, and raise your arms slightly behind you.

6

Twist your torso to the right, lowering your right shoulder and arm. Keep your back straight.

7

Twist your torso to the left, lowering your left shoulder and arm. Twist 12 times in each direction.

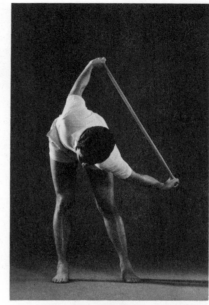

8

Stand up straight and bring the dowel back to its original position in front of you. Again, bend your arms only if you must.

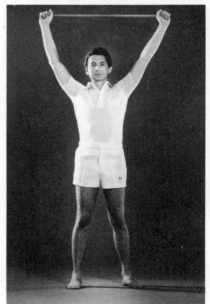

AIR CYCLING

"Bicycling" in the air is a standard and effective exercise for trimming the midriff and shows results quickly. If it causes any back pain, however, consult your doctor before continuing.

To Reduce: repeat sequence 4 times

Maintenance: repeat sequence 8 times

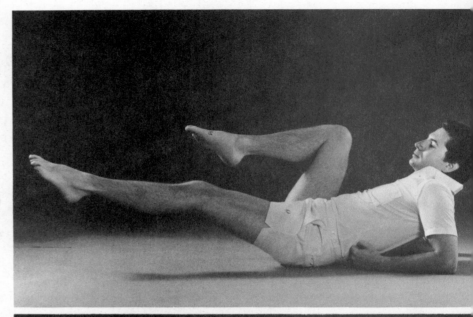

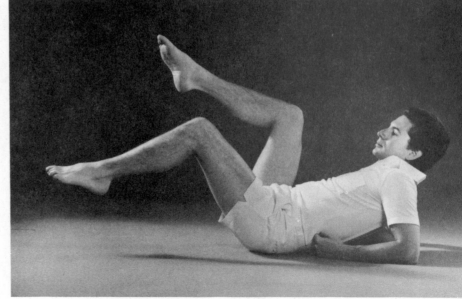

1

Lie on the floor with your torso propped up on your elbows. Your legs should be straight, feet together and pointed, and your forearms parallel to your body. Bend your right knee and bring it up to your chest.

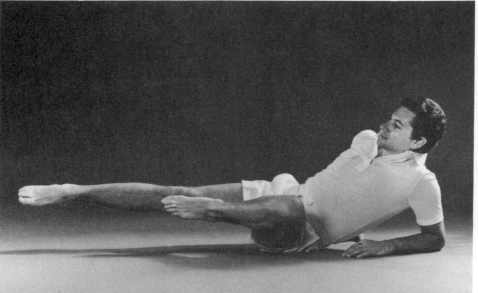

3

Lean onto the left side of your fanny and pedal 8 times with each leg; then lean onto the right side and pedal 8 more times with each leg.

2

Straighten and lower your right leg to within 6 inches of the floor and bend your left knee to your chest. Straighten your left leg and lower it to within 6 inches of the floor while you bend your right knee to your chest. This should resemble pedaling a bicycle. Make 8 pedaling motions with each leg.

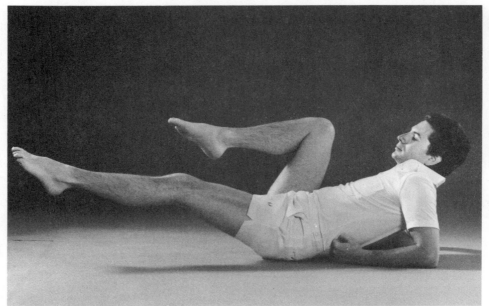

4

Return to the original position and make the cycling motions 8 final times with each leg.

UP, UP AND AROUND

This exercise is strenuous, but you'll find it works effectively to reduce your paunch. If it causes any back pain, altering the exercise by making small arcs with your legs and keeping them higher off the floor may eliminate the discomfort. Check with your doctor if pain continues.

To Reduce: repeat sequence 4 times from step 2

Maintenance: add 4 times a week, working up to 20

208

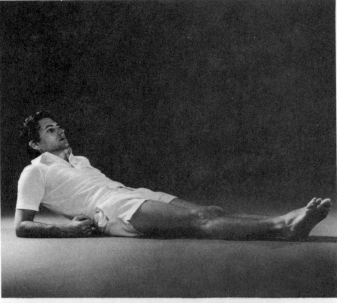

1

Lie on the floor with your torso propped up on your elbows. Your legs should be straight, feet together and pointed, and your forearms should be parallel to your body.

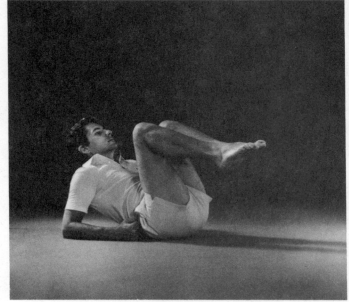

2

Bend both legs, bringing the knees up to your chest. Keep your stomach muscles tightened.

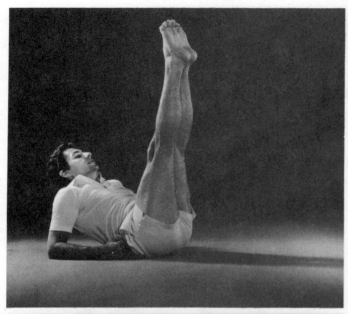

3

Straighten both legs so they are perpendicular to the floor. Do not rock back on your shoulders.

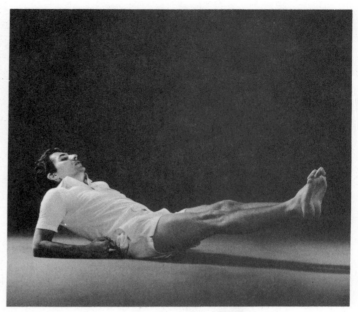

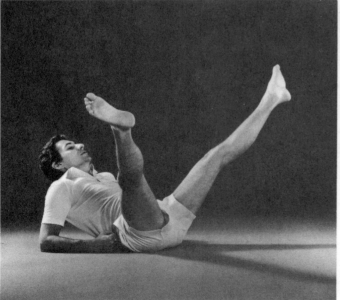

4

Making wide arcs with each leg, begin to lower them slowly without bending your knees.

5

When your legs are about 10 inches from the floor, bring them together. Hold this position for 2 seconds, keeping your knees straight and your stomach tightened. Bring your knees up to your chest, as in step 2, and repeat.

MILITARY TOE TOUCH

If you can't touch the floor, reach for your shins until you're more flexible. Be careful not to strain your lower back as you bend over, and keep your knees straight.

To Reduce: repeat sequence 16 times

Maintenance: repeat sequence 24 times

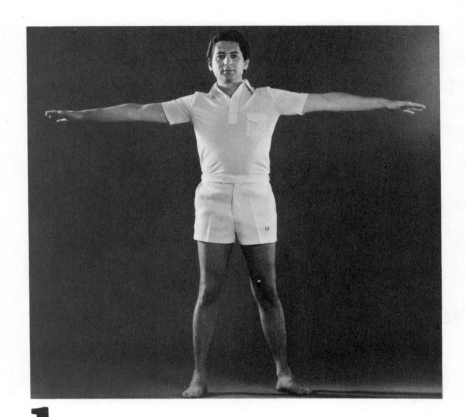

1

Stand with your legs straight, feet apart, and arms stretched out to the side at shoulder height.

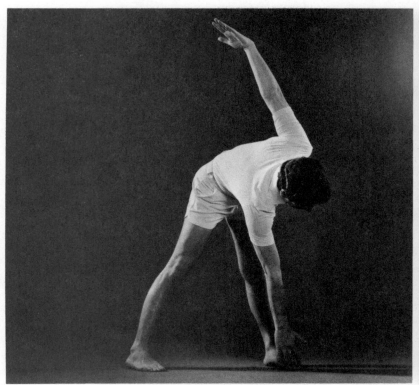

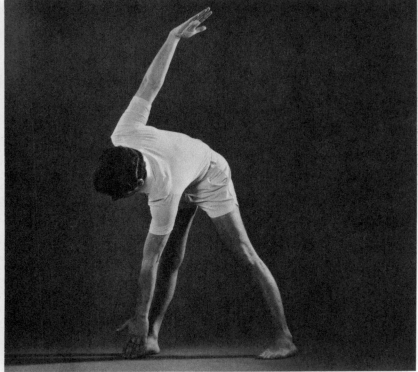

2

Keeping your legs straight, bend forward from the hips and touch your left foot with your right hand. Your left arm should be stretched back above your head.

3

Return to the original position with your arms stretched out straight. Bend forward again and touch your right foot with your left hand, stretching your right arm above your head.

PECKING

When you finish this exercise, unclasp your hands and grab your calves, then slowly pull your torso toward your shins. Hold this position for 4 seconds, then relax; this will loosen your muscles.

To Reduce: repeat sequence 5 times

Maintenance: the same

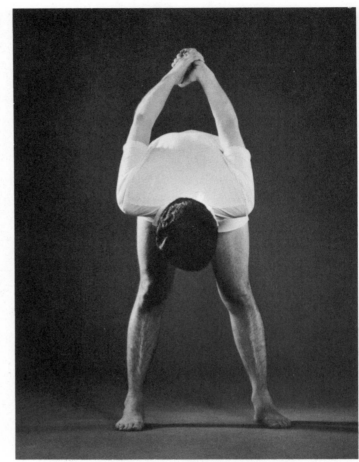

1

Stand with your legs straight, feet apart, and torso bent forward from the hips. Clasp your hands behind your back and raise them as high as you can. Keeping your legs straight, bounce your torso toward the floor 8 times.

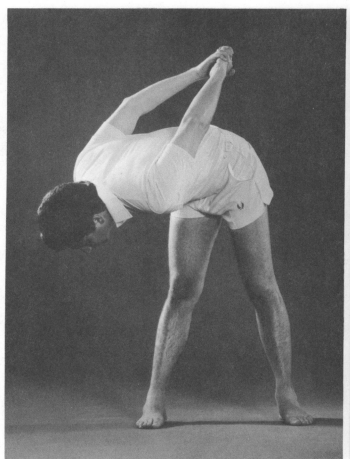

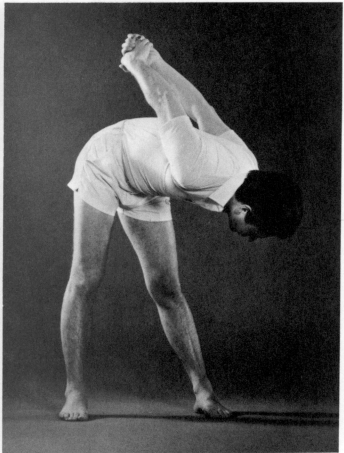

2

Lean your torso over
your right leg and bounce
8 times, keeping your
arms raised behind your
back.

3

Lean your torso over
your left leg and bounce 8
more times. Return to
the forward position and
bounce 8 final times.

ON YOUR MARK

This exercise will strengthen the fronts of your thighs and stretch the muscles all along your legs.

To Reduce: repeat sequence 8 times

Maintenance: repeat sequence 12 times

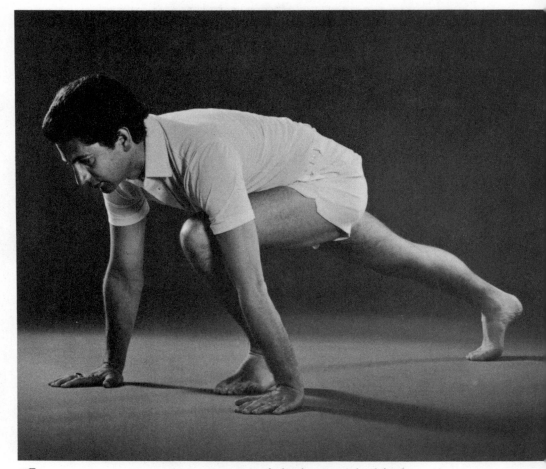

1

Starting in a "get-set" position, on the balls of your feet with your hands flat on the floor and your arms straight, stretch your right leg out behind you. Your left leg should be bent, with the knee between your arms.

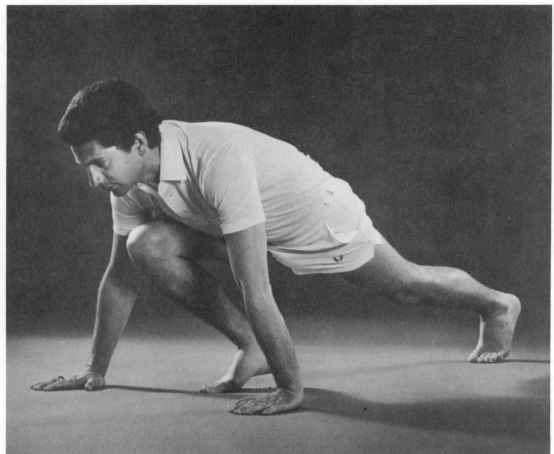

2

Keeping your hands on the floor and moving your back as little as possible, push off your feet and switch the position of your legs. Your left leg should now be stretched out behind and your right leg bent between your arms. Jump back to the original position.

AROUND THE CLOCK

Be careful not to arch your back or stick out your fanny while you do this exercise. Keep your stomach and fanny muscles tightened.

To Reduce: repeat sequence 4 times

Maintenance: repeat sequence 8 times

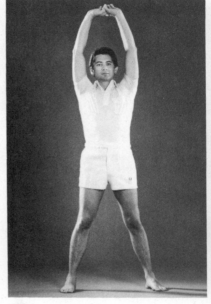

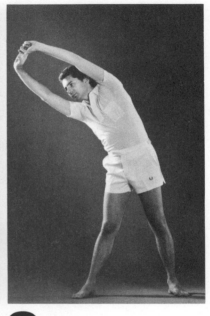

1

Stand with your legs straight, feet slightly apart, and arms stretched straight up in the air. Clasp your hands above your head, palms facing up, and tighten your stomach and fanny muscles.

2

Slowly stretch your arms to the right without bending forward at the waist. Your body should form an arc.

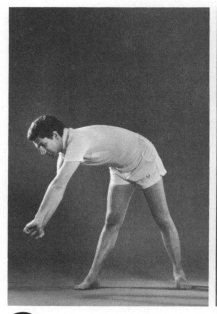

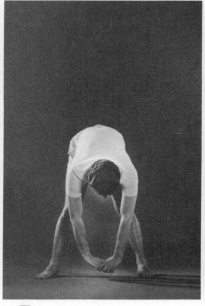

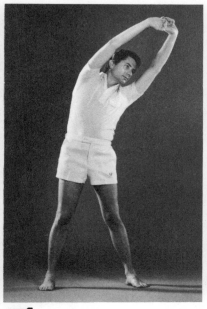

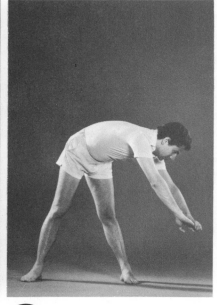

3

Twist your torso
to the right so
your chest is
parallel to
the floor.
Continue the
circular motion
of your body,
lowering your
hands.

4

Bring your torso
around so your
arms hang in
front of you.

5

Raise your
clasped hands up
to the left,
making an arc as
you did in step 2,
and return to the
original position.

6

Reverse
directions and
stretch your
arms and torso
to the left, then
continue to make a
counterclockwise
circle with your body.

MAINTENANCE PROGRAMS

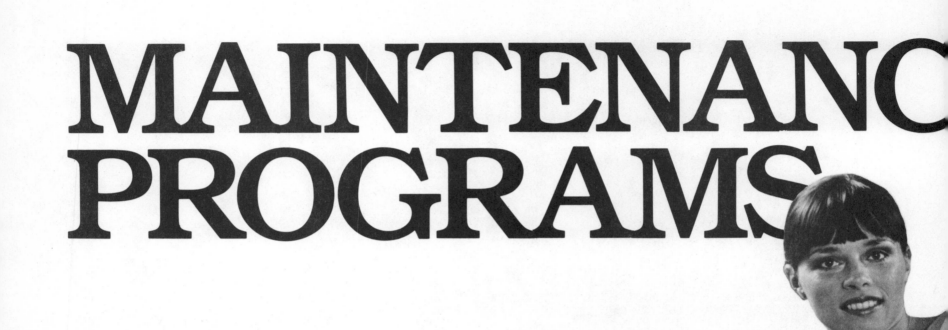

After three weeks of spot reducing, when improvements have become apparent, you should begin the appropriate maintenance routines. Though the repetitions will increase, you can actually do fewer exercises. Performance of the maintenance routines will continue to help you develop the body you have always wanted. Perform the repetitions regularly, and you will maintain the results you have already achieved. Don't forget that the flexibility exercises are an important part of your spot reducing program. You should conclude each of your sessions with the recommended stretching exercises.

ARMS, STOMACH, BREASTS, WAIST AND MIDRIFF

ALWAYS END WITH THE FOLLOWING FLEXIBILITY EXERCISES:

ARMS, SHOULDERS, WAIST AND MIDRIFF, STOMACH, HIPS, AND FANNY

ALWAYS END WITH THE FOLLOWING FLEXIBILITY EXERCISES:

WAIST AND MIDRIFF, STOMACH, HIPS, FANNY AND THIGHS

ALWAYS END WITH THE FOLLOWING FLEXIBILITY EXERCISES:

STOMACH, HIPS, FANNY AND THIGHS

ALWAYS END WITH THE FOLLOWING FLEXIBILITY EXERCISES:

HIPS, FANNY, THIGHS, CALVES AND ANKLES

ALWAYS END WITH THE FOLLOWING FLEXIBILITY EXERCISES:

ARMS, STOMACH, FANNY AND THIGHS

ALWAYS END WITH THE FOLLOWING FLEXIBILITY EXERCISES:

FOR THE WHOLE BODY

ALWAYS END WITH THE FOLLOWING FLEXIBILITY EXERCISES: